GASTROINTESTINAL CANCER CARE
FOR ONCOLOGY NURSES

Edited by
Lisa Parks, MS, ANP-BC, and
Meghan M. Findlay, MSN, GNP/ANP, AOCNP®

Oncology Nursing Society
Pittsburgh, Pennsylvania

ONS Publications Department
Publisher and Director of Publications: William A. Tony, BA, CQIA
Senior Editorial Manager: Lisa M. George, BA
Assistant Editorial Manager: Amy Nicoletti, BA, JD
Acquisitions Editor: John Zaphyr, BA, MEd
Associate Staff Editors: Casey S. Kennedy, BA, Andrew Petyak, BA
Design and Production Administrator: Dany Sjoen
Editorial Assistant: Judy Holmes

Copyright © 2019 by the Oncology Nursing Society. All rights reserved. No part of the material protected by this copyright may be reproduced or utilized in any form, electronic or mechanical, including photocopying, recording, or by an information storage and retrieval system, without written permission from the copyright owner. For information, visit www.ons.org/sites/default/files/Publication%20Permissions.pdf, or send an email to pubpermissions@ons.org.

Library of Congress Cataloging-in-Publication Data

Names: Parks, Lisa, 1958- editor. | Findlay, Meghan M., editor. | Oncology Nursing Society, issuing body.
Title: Gastrointestinal cancer care for oncology nurses / edited by Lisa Parks and Meghan M. Findlay.
Description: Pittsburgh, Pennsylvania : Oncology Nursing Society, [2019] | Includes bibliographical references and index.
Identifiers: LCCN 2018033803 (print) | LCCN 2018034956 (ebook) | ISBN 9781635930290 (ebook) | ISBN 9781635930283
Subjects: | MESH: Gastrointestinal Neoplasms–nursing | Oncology Nursing–methods
Classification: LCC RD668.3 (ebook) | LCC RD668.3 (print) | NLM WY 156 | DDC 616.99/4330231–dc23
LC record available at https://lccn.loc.gov/2018033803

Publisher's Note

This book is published by the Oncology Nursing Society (ONS). ONS neither represents nor guarantees that the practices described herein will, if followed, ensure safe and effective patient care. The recommendations contained in this book reflect ONS's judgment regarding the state of general knowledge and practice in the field as of the date of publication. The recommendations may not be appropriate for use in all circumstances. Those who use this book should make their own determinations regarding specific safe and appropriate patient care practices, taking into account the personnel, equipment, and practices available at the hospital or other facility at which they are located. The editors and publisher cannot be held responsible for any liability incurred as a consequence from the use or application of any of the contents of this book. Figures and tables are used as examples only. They are not meant to be all-inclusive, nor do they represent endorsement of any particular institution by ONS. Mention of specific products and opinions related to those products do not indicate or imply endorsement by ONS. Websites mentioned are provided for information only; the hosts are responsible for their own content and availability. Unless otherwise indicated, dollar amounts reflect U.S. dollars.

ONS publications are originally published in English. Publishers wishing to translate ONS publications must contact ONS about licensing arrangements. ONS publications cannot be translated without obtaining written permission from ONS. (Individual tables and figures that are reprinted or adapted require additional permission from the original source.) Because translations from English may not always be accurate or precise, ONS disclaims any responsibility for inaccuracies in words or meaning that may occur as a result of the translation. Readers relying on precise information should check the original English version.

Printed in the United States of America

Innovation • Excellence • Advocacy

Contributors

Editors

Lisa Parks, MS, ANP-BC
Hepatobiliary Nurse Practitioner
Division of Surgical Oncology
The Ohio State University James Cancer Hospital and Solove Research Institute
Columbus, Ohio
Chapter 3. Gastric Cancer

Meghan M. Findlay, MSN, GNP/ANP, AOCNP®
PhD Candidate
University of Utah
Salt Lake City, Utah

Authors

Jessica MacIntyre, ARNP, NP-C, AOCNP®
Nurse Practitioner
University of Miami Sylvester Comprehensive Cancer Center
Miami, Florida
Chapter 4. Pancreatic Cancer; Chapter 6. Primary Liver and Biliary Tract Cancers; Chapter 7. Small Bowel Cancer

Steve Malangone, MSN, FNP-C, AOCNP®
Nurse Practitioner
University of Arizona Cancer Center
Tucson, Arizona
Chapter 1. Colon, Rectal, and Anal Cancers

Laura A. Pachella, RN, MSN, AGPCNP-BC, AOCNP®
Advanced Practice Registered Nurse
University of Texas MD Anderson Cancer Center
Houston, Texas
Chapter 2. Esophageal Cancer

Cheryl Pfennig, MSN, RN, NP-C, AOCNP®
Advanced Practice Registered Nurse
Department of Surgical Oncology
University of Texas MD Anderson Cancer Center
Houston, Texas
Chapter 3. Gastric Cancer

Pamela Ryan, BSN, RN, ONN-CG
Manager, Neuroendocrine Tumor Program
Ochsner Medical Center–Kenner
Kenner, Louisiana
Chapter 5. Neuroendocrine Cancers

Amber Thomassen, MA, MSN, APRN-BC, AOCNP®
Phase I/ET Nurse Practitioner
University of Miami Sylvester Comprehensive Cancer Center
Miami, Florida
Chapter 7. Small Bowel Cancer

Brianne Voros, MS
Research Associate, Neuroendocrine Tumor Program
Department of Surgery, Louisiana State University Health Sciences Center
New Orleans, Louisiana
Chapter 5. Neuroendocrine Cancers

Disclosure

Editors and authors of books and guidelines provided by the Oncology Nursing Society are expected to disclose to the readers any significant financial interest or other relationships with the manufacturer(s) of any commercial products.

A vested interest may be considered to exist if a contributor is affiliated with or has a financial interest in commercial organizations that may have a direct or indirect interest in the subject matter. A "financial interest" may include, but is not limited to, being a shareholder in the organization; being an employee of the commercial organization; serving on an organization's speakers bureau; or receiving research funding from the organization. An "affiliation" may be holding a position on an advisory board or some other role of benefit to the commercial organization. Vested interest statements appear in the front matter for each publication.

Contributors are expected to disclose any unlabeled or investigational use of products discussed in their content. This information is acknowledged solely for the information of the readers.

The contributors provided the following disclosure and vested interest information:

Jessica MacIntyre, ARNP, NP-C, AOCNP®: Celgene Corp., Genentech, Inc., honoraria

Pamela Ryan, BSN, RN, ONN-CG: Ipsen, consultant or advisory role, honoraria, research funding

Table of Contents

Preface vii

Chapter 1. Colon, Rectal, and Anal Cancers 1
    Introduction 1
    Incidence and Epidemiology 2
    Etiology and Risk Factors 3
    Signs and Symptoms 6
    Diagnostic Evaluation 6
    Treatment 9
    Nursing Care 19
    Prognosis 21
    Prevention 22
    High-Risk Assessment: Screening and Genetic Testing 23
    Surveillance 25
    Survivorship 26
    Summary 28
    References 29

Chapter 2. Esophageal Cancer 39
    Introduction 39
    Anatomy of the Esophagus 39
    Incidence and Epidemiology 42
    Etiology and Risk Factors 42
    Signs and Symptoms 44
    Diagnostic Evaluation 45
    Clinical Staging 46
    Treatment 47
    Nursing Care 56
    Prognosis 59
    Prevention 60
    High-Risk Assessment: Screening and Genetic Testing 61
    Surveillance 62
    Survivorship 62
    Comparison of Esophageal and Gastric Cancers 64

    Summary 65
    References 66

Chapter 3. Gastric Cancer 71
    Introduction 71
    Incidence and Epidemiology 71
    Etiology and Risk Factors 71
    Signs and Symptoms 73
    Diagnostic Evaluation 74
    Treatment 76
    Nursing Care 85
    Prognosis 86
    Prevention 87
    Surveillance 87
    Survivorship 88
    Summary 89
    References 89

Chapter 4. Pancreatic Cancer 95
    Introduction 95
    Incidence and Epidemiology 95
    Etiology and Risk Factors 95
    Signs and Symptoms 97
    Diagnostic Evaluation 98
    Treatment 101
    Nursing Care 106
    Prognosis 106
    Prevention 107
    Surveillance 107
    Survivorship 107
    Summary 108
    References 109

Chapter 5. Neuroendocrine Cancers 111
    Introduction 111
    Incidence and Epidemiology 112
    Etiology and Risk Factors 113
    Signs and Symptoms 113

Diagnostic Evaluation............................ 120
Histology and Staging........................ 123
Treatment 125
Nursing Care 131
Prevention 134
Prognosis 134
Surveillance 134
Survivorship 134
Summary.. 135
References... 135

Chapter 6. Primary Liver and Biliary Tract Cancers........................ 141
Introduction 141
Primary Liver Cancer 142
Biliary Tract Cancers: Cholangiocarcinoma and Gallbladder Cancer......................... 157
Summary.. 170
References... 170

Chapter 7. Small Bowel Cancer 175
Introduction 175
Incidence and Epidemiology 175
Etiology and Risk Factors 175
Signs and Symptoms........................... 177
Diagnostic Evaluation......................... 178
Histology 179
Clinical Staging..................................... 179
Prognosis 180
Treatment 181
Nursing Care 183
Prevention 183
Surveillance 184
Survivorship 184
Summary.. 184
References... 185

Index... 187

Preface

Gastrointestinal cancers account for more deaths worldwide than any other cancers. Surgical resection is the primary curative treatment for these cancers, but unfortunately, the majority of cancers are surgically unresectable at the time of diagnosis. Pancreatic and biliary tract cancers still have unknown biology, which has prevented the development of targeted agents for their treatment. Radiation therapy and neoadjuvant or adjuvant chemotherapy have not had a large impact on overall survival rates.

Immunotherapy is an emerging option for gastrointestinal cancer treatment. This therapy directly targets T cells, not tumor antigens. Immunotherapy drugs can overcome immune resistance and produce tumor response. Cancer vaccines, a form of immunotherapy, work by activating T cells for immunity. These T cells can then produce cell cytotoxicity.

With increased endoscopic surveillance and radiologic imaging, progress has been made in earlier detection of gastrointestinal cancers and premalignant lesions, especially in colon cancer. However, some individuals at high risk for developing colon cancer do not participate in recommended screenings. Vaccination against hepatitis B and C in high-risk groups, as well as treatment for *Helicobacter pylori*, could decrease the incidence of gastrointestinal cancers.

Oncology nurses know cancer treatment is constantly evolving. Awareness of current prevention and screening strategies for gastrointestinal cancers is imperative. Oncology nurses must have knowledge of gastrointestinal cancers and treatment strategies to provide patients with personalized care and education. The editors offer this text as a reference for the nursing care of patients with gastrointestinal cancer.

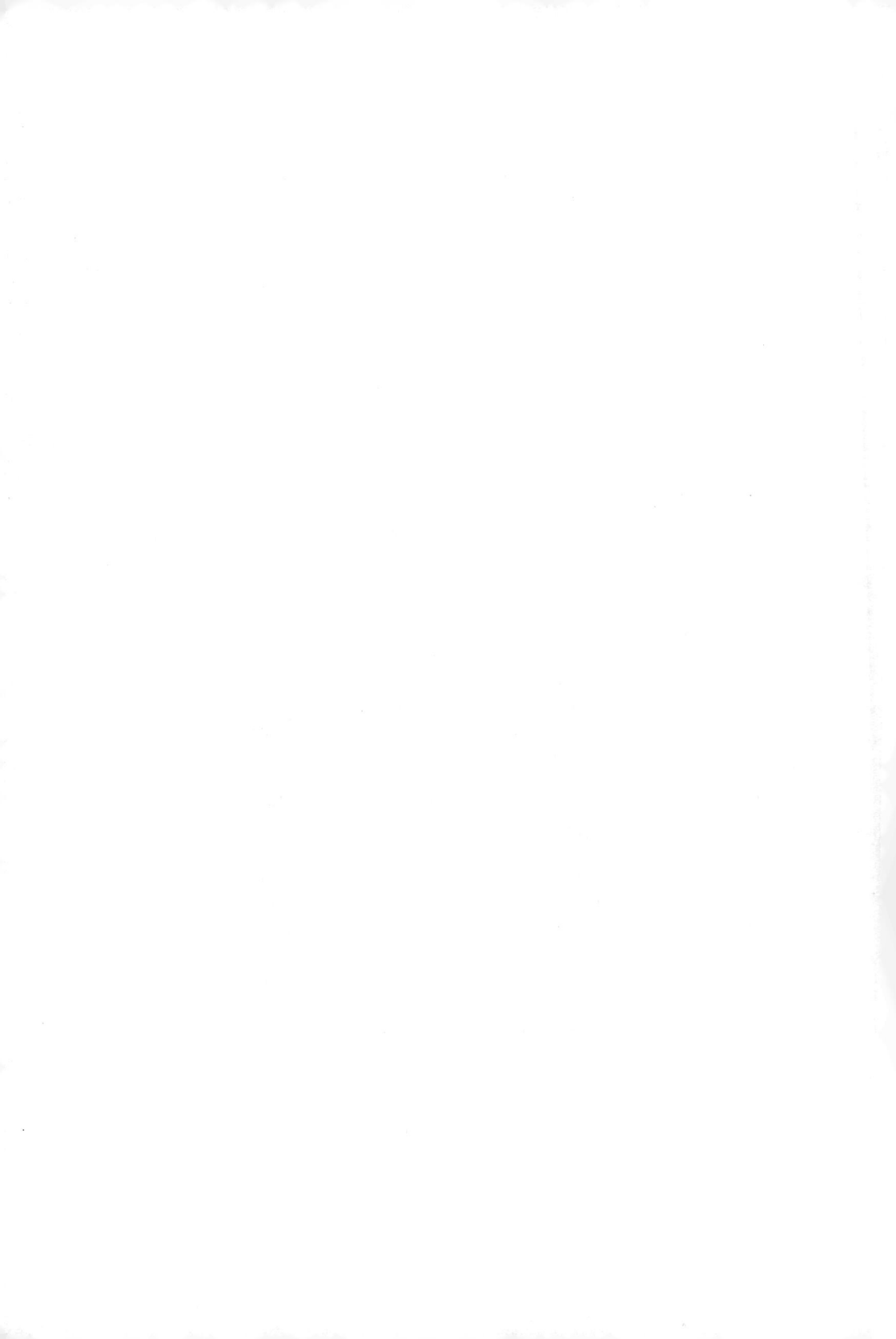

CHAPTER 1

Colon, Rectal, and Anal Cancers

Steve Malangone, MSN, FNP-C, AOCNP®

Introduction

Colorectal adenocarcinoma is an epithelial-derived cancer that arises from the colonic mucosa. More than 90% of colorectal cancers arise from adenomatous polyps (Levin et al., 2008). On the cellular level, the transformation of normal colonic mucosa to invasive cancer occurs over a decade or longer, with an identified multistep progression from normal colonic mucosa to adenomatous polyp to invasive cancer (Sagiv et al., 2006). This process is associated with defined, albeit heterogeneous, genetic events (Pino & Chung, 2010). Once invasive biology occurs, colorectal adenocarcinoma can invade both locally through direct invasion and distantly through lymphatic and hematogenous spread.

The location of the tumor in the colorectum (see Figure 1-1) has therapeutic and prognostic relevance. Tumors located in the rectum, defined as below the peritoneal reflection (typically, the 12–15 cm above the anal verge), are classified as rectal cancer, whereas tumors located above the peritoneal reflection are classified as colon cancer (Kenig & Richter, 2013). In comparison to colon cancer, rectal cancer is associated with a relatively high rate of local recurrence, resulting in considerable morbidity and mortality (Sauer et al., 2004). This critical distinction in diagnosis is needed to identify a proper interprofessional management strategy (see Preoperative Management).

Anal cancer represents a less common form of gastrointestinal malignancy that arises from the epithelium of the anal canal. Anal cancers are distinct from rectal cancers and perianal skin cancers in that they originate from the epithelium between the anorectal ring and the anal verge (Czito, Ahmed, Kalady, & Eng, 2015). Anal cancer epidemiology, risk factors, prognosis, and histology represent a distinct entity and are discussed in the following sections.

Figure 1-1. Colorectal Cancer

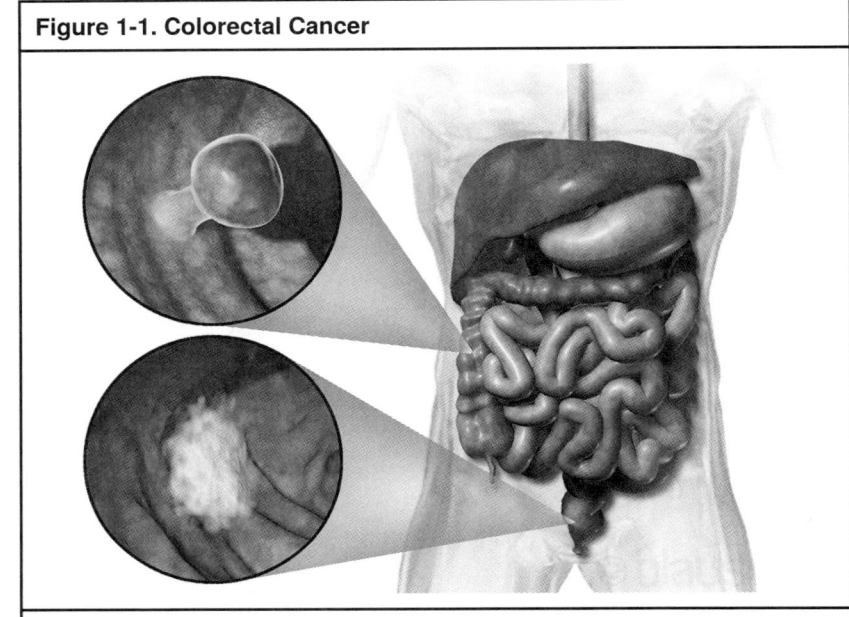

Note. Image courtesy of Blausen Medical Communications, Inc., via Wikimedia Commons. Retrieved from https://commons.wikimedia.org/wiki/File:Blausen_0246_ColorectalCancer.png. Used under the Creative Commons Attribution 3.0 Unported (CC BY 3.0) license (https://creativecommons.org/licenses/by/3.0/legalcode).

Incidence and Epidemiology

The lifetime risk of developing colorectal cancer in the United States is estimated at 5% (Siegel, Miller, & Jemal, 2018). As the fourth most frequently diagnosed cancer for both sexes combined, colorectal cancer is a common malignancy, with 140,250 new cases estimated for 2018 in the United States. It is also the second leading cause of cancer death for both sexes combined (Siegel et al., 2018).

Colorectal cancer represents significant morbidity and mortality globally. The estimated global incidence is 1.4 million new cases per year, with approximately 694,000 deaths estimated annually (Torre et al., 2015).

Overall, colorectal cancer incidence in the United States is declining. Between 2005 and 2014, incidence declined 3% per year (Siegel et al., 2018). This decrease is attributable to relative reduction in risk factors and increased use of screening colonoscopy with removal of precancerous polyps (Siegel, Ward, & Jemal, 2012).

In contrast, colorectal cancer incidence is rising among people younger than age 50 in the United States. From the mid-1980s through

2013, colon and rectal cancer rates in adults aged 20–29 years and 40–54 years increased at an annual rate of 1%–2.4% and 0.5%–1.3%, respectively. Rectal cancer in people younger than age 55 now represents one-third of all new diagnoses, with a disproportionately higher increase of 3.2% annually from 1974 to 2013 in the 20–29-year age group. The proportion of rectal cancer cases in people younger than age 55 in the United States has doubled in the past three decades, from 14.6% to 29.2% (Siegel et al., 2017). Familial syndromes account for approximately 20% of these cases while 80% are sporadic (Ahnen et al., 2014). Young-onset colorectal cancers occur more frequently in the distal colon and rectum and are more likely to be poorly differentiated, have signet ring features, and present at advanced stages compared with those diagnosed at a later onset (Ahnen et al., 2014).

Mortality from colorectal cancer is decreasing in the United States. Mortality decreased by 35% from 1990 to 2007 (Henley et al., 2015) and by 50% from 1970 to 2015 (Siegel et al., 2018). This trend is attributable to earlier detection and improved therapies (Jemal et al., 2011).

Anal cancer is a relatively uncommon malignancy, with 8,580 new cases estimated for 2018 in the United States (Siegel et al., 2018). Despite the rarity of anal cancer, the incidence has almost doubled in recent years, from 1.2 cases per 100,000 per year during 1973–1996 to 2.2 cases per 100,000 per year during 1997–2009 (Nelson, Levine, Bernstein, Smith, & Lai, 2013). The increased rates result from increased risk factors, including infection with oncogenic human papillomavirus (HPV), immunocompromised conditions, and smoking.

Etiology and Risk Factors

Modifiable and nonmodifiable risk factors contribute to the development of colorectal adenocarcinoma. Several clearly defined familial syndromes have been identified, the most common of which are familial adenomatous polyposis, hereditary nonpolyposis colorectal cancer (also known as Lynch syndrome), Peutz-Jeghers syndrome, and juvenile polyposis syndrome (Burt & Neklason, 2005; see Table 1-1).

The National Comprehensive Cancer Network® (NCCN®, 2018d) recommends that whenever possible, patients with a significant family history of colorectal or associated cancer, a known family history of familial cancer syndrome, or a history of multiple cancer primaries be referred to a genetic counselor. The purpose of this referral is for review of history, consideration of germline genetic testing, and provision of screening recommendations for patients and potentially affected family members.

Table 1-1. Familial Syndromes Associated With Increased Risk for Colorectal Cancer

Syndrome	Prevalence	Clinical Features	Lifetime Risk of Developing Colorectal Cancer	Genes Involved	Screening and Treatment Recommendations
Familial adenomatous polyposis (FAP)	< 1% of all colorectal cases	> 10–20 polyps, often associated with 100s to 1,000s of colonic polyps; also associated with desmoid tumor, hepatoblastoma, and thyroid cancer	100% in classic FAP	APC (adenomatous polyposis coli) MUTYH	Referral to genetics; referral to surgery for consideration of total proctocolectomy
Hereditary nonpolyposis colorectal cancer (Lynch syndrome)	3%–5% of all colorectal cancer cases	Not associated with polyposis; strong family history of colorectal, endometrial, and urothelial malignancy	50%–80% (MLH1, MSH2) 15%–20% (MSH6) 10%–22% (PMS2)	Mismatch repair genes: MLH1, MSH2, MSH6, PMS2	Referral to genetics
Juvenile polyposis syndrome	Rare; < 1% of all colorectal cancer cases	Autosomal dominant, strong family history, right-sided hamartomatous polyps, rectal bleeding is common	50%	BMPR1A MADH4	Referral to genetics
Peutz-Jeghers syndrome	Rare; < 1% of all colorectal cancer cases	Personal or family history of breast, colorectal, small intestine, pancreatic, ovarian, and lung cancers	39%	STK11 (LKB1)	Referral to genetics

Note. Based on information from Burt & Neklason, 2005; National Comprehensive Cancer Network, 2018c.

Inflammatory bowel disease, including Crohn disease and ulcerative colitis, is associated with a risk approximately six times that of the general population's risk of developing colorectal cancer (Ekbom, Helmick, Zack, & Adami, 1990). Because of the high risk for developing colorectal cancer, earlier and more frequent endoscopic surveillance is recommended in patients with inflammatory bowel disease (Rutter, 2011).

Environmental modifiable factors play a significant role in the etiologic development of colorectal cancer. Inactivity, a diet high in red and processed meats, and a diet high in refined starches and sugars are related to increased risk of colorectal cancer (Chan & Giovannucci, 2010). This is demonstrated in the highly variable global patterns of prevalence. Regions following a Western lifestyle, such as Australia and New Zealand, Europe, and North America, show the highest rates of colorectal cancer (35–45 cases per 100,000 per year), compared with regions not following a Western lifestyle, such as Africa, Eastern Asia, and Eastern Europe (3–14 cases per 100,000 per year), which show the lowest rates (Jemal et al., 2011).

Diets high in red and processed meats have been associated with significantly higher rates of colorectal cancer, especially after high-temperature cooking (Martinez et al., 2007). The exact mechanism for this increased risk is unknown, but a hypothesis includes increased exposure of the colonic mucosa to mutagenic substances (Chan & Giovannucci, 2010). Obesity is a correlative risk factor, with higher levels of obesity showing higher correlative risk of developing colorectal cancer (Karahalios, English, & Simpson, 2015). Vitamin D deficiency also is associated with increased risk of developing colorectal cancer (Chung, Lee, Terasawa, Lau, & Trikalinos, 2011).

Colonic polyps are the premalignant precursor to colorectal cancer in at least 90% of cases (Libutti, Saltz, Willett, & Levine, 2015). A personal history of large (larger than 1 cm) tubulovillous, villous, or adenomatous polyps is associated with a higher risk for developing subsequent colorectal adenocarcinoma, whereas polyps smaller than 1 cm are not associated with higher risk (Libutti et al., 2015).

Family history of colorectal adenocarcinoma is associated with increased risk for developing colorectal cancer. Having a single first-degree relative with a history of colorectal adenocarcinoma is associated with approximately double the risk, with further increases in risk as the number of first- and second-degree relatives with colorectal cancer increases (Taylor, Burt, Williams, Haug, & Cannon-Albright, 2010).

The risk factors for developing anal cancer are etiologically distinct from those for developing colorectal cancer. The most significant risk factor for the development of anal cancer is chronic infection with oncogenic strains of HPV, which has been identified in up to 88% of anal squamous cell tumors (Daling et al., 2004). Etiologically, chronic infection with oncogenic HPV type 16 is associated with the development of premalignant dysplastic changes analogous to those seen in cervical cancers. These lesions, termed *high-grade intraepithelial neoplasia*, progress further to undergo malignant transformation (Czito et al., 2015). Additional associated risk factors include chronic immunosuppression, HIV infection, and cigarette smoking (Daling et al., 2004; Frisch, 2000).

Signs and Symptoms

In the early stage, colorectal adenocarcinoma rarely causes significant symptoms. Colonoscopic surveillance, when performed as recommended, can identify and cure the majority of early colonic neoplasms (Brenner, Chang-Claude, Seiler, Stürmer, & Hoffmeister, 2007). Unfortunately, despite improvements in screening colonoscopy use, the majority of colorectal cancers are diagnosed at a more advanced stage: when symptoms develop (Moreno et al., 2016). In more advanced disease, these symptoms include abdominal pain, change in bowel habits, iron-deficiency anemia, hematochezia, melena, and colonic obstruction (Hamilton, Round, Sharp, & Peters, 2005). Additionally, 20% of colorectal adenocarcinoma is diagnosed after development of metastatic disease, and in these cases, symptoms secondary to metastatic sites, such as jaundice secondary to biliary obstruction from liver metastases, can be the presenting symptom (Kanas et al., 2012).

The most common presenting symptom of anal cancer is bleeding; other common symptoms include pain, pruritus, and change in bowel pattern (Hamilton et al., 2005). Patients often self-treat for presumed hemorrhoid-related symptoms, thus delaying seeking medical attention until self-treatment fails. Frequently, patients and healthcare providers mistakenly attribute these symptoms to benign anal conditions such as hemorrhoids or anal fissures, which also may be coexistent. Unfortunately, the delay from symptom onset to diagnosis is common, ranging from two weeks to more than four years and averaging six months (Czito et al., 2015).

Diagnostic Evaluation

Evaluation of colorectal adenocarcinoma includes the patient's medical history, family history, physical assessment, and laboratory analysis of complete blood count, renal and hepatic function, and measurement of carcinoembryonic antigen (CEA). To assess the extent of local disease and evaluate for the presence of distant disease, imaging of the chest, abdomen, and pelvis with either computed tomography (CT) or magnetic resonance imaging is also indicated (Libutti et al., 2015). A tissue sample is used to establish a diagnosis and evaluate for molecular and genetic markers. It is typically obtained during colonoscopy but may be obtained surgically in the event of an urgent indication for resection, such as colonic perforation. Colonoscopy is also needed to differentiate colon versus rectal cancer, which has therapeutic implications, and to evaluate for synchronous (more than one) primaries, which are present in approximately 4% of cases (Mulder et al., 2011; Sauer et al., 2004).

The diagnosis of anal cancer can be initially made on rectal examination and typically is identified as an intraluminal mass. For painful lesions, examination under anesthesia is performed, with incisional biopsy required to establish pathologic diagnosis. Palpation of inguinal lymph nodes is also performed, with fine needle aspiration of any enlarged inguinal lymph nodes to assess for local lymph node involvement (Czito et al., 2015). Once diagnosis is confirmed, advanced imaging with CT of the chest and abdomen, as well as magnetic resonance imaging of the pelvis, is recommended to assess for the extent of local disease and evaluate for the presence of metastatic disease. Positron-emission tomography may offer additional sensitivity in identification of lymph node metastases that may not be found with CT alone (Jones, Hruby, Solomon, Rutherford, & Martin, 2015).

Histology

Colorectal adenocarcinoma arises from gland-forming epithelium. The degree of differentiation is related to the degree of gland formation on histologic examination at the cellular level, with poorly differentiated tumors being associated with worse prognosis (Compton et al., 2000). Mucinous adenocarcinomas are a histologic subtype associated with increase in intracellular and extracellular mucin, which is associated with a higher likelihood of peritoneal and lymphatic spread and a poorer prognosis overall (Kanemitsu et al., 2003). Carcinomas that have a predominant accumulation of mucin within the cell are classified as signet ring cell carcinomas. Signet ring cell carcinomas represent an uncommon, very aggressive variant associated with significantly lower rates of survival (Libutti et al., 2015). Invasion into the lymphatic, perineural, and vascular space also is assessed upon standard pathologic review. Tumors that invade the lymphovascular space are associated with more invasive disease in general and poorer five-year survival (Lim et al., 2010). Perineural invasion also confers poorer prognosis, with approximately double the rates of metastatic recurrence when present (Knijn, Mogk, Teerenstra, Simmer, & Nagtegaal, 2016).

Anal cancers arise from the epithelium of the anal canal and are predominantly of squamous cell histology. Less commonly, glandular cells of the anal canal may lead to adenocarcinomas, which are associated with a biology and treatment paradigm most similar to rectal adenocarcinoma. Pathologic specimens associated with chronic HPV infection may be stained for p16, which is a marker for HPV infection identified in the majority of cases of anal squamous cell carcinoma (Serup-Hansen et al., 2014).

Clinical Staging

Both colon and rectal adenocarcinoma are staged using the American Joint Committee on Cancer (AJCC) tumor-node-metastasis, or TNM, staging system (Jessup et al., 2017). The *T* stage defines the extent of the primary tumor, *N* designates the number of regional lymph nodes, and *M* denotes the presence of metastatic disease (Jessup et al., 2017). T1 invasion is defined as involving the submucosa; T2 as penetration through the submucosa into the muscularis propria; T3 as penetration through the muscularis propria into the pericolorectal tissues; T4a as penetration into the visceral peritoneum; and T4b as directly invading adjacent organs. Regional lymph nodes are classified by *N*, with N0 indicating no lymph node involvement. N1 is classified as metastasis in one to three regional lymph nodes and is further divided into N1a, N1b, and N1c. N1a describes metastasis in one lymph node. N1b designates two to three lymph nodes, whereas N1c denotes tumoral deposits in the pericolonic tissue. N2 is defined as metastasis in four or more lymph nodes, with N2a and N2b describing metastasis in four to six regional lymph nodes and seven or more lymph nodes, respectively. M1 designation indicates the presence of distant metastatic disease, with M1a describing metastasis in one site or organ without peritoneal metastasis, M1b as metastasis to two more sites without peritoneal metastasis, and M1c as metastasis to the peritoneal surface. Stage I disease includes T1 or T2, lymph node–negative, nonmetastatic disease. Stage IIA, IIB, and IIIC disease includes T3–T4, lymph node–negative, nonmetastatic disease. Stage IIIA, IIIB, and IIIC disease includes lymph node–positive, nonmetastatic disease, and stage IVA, IVB, and IVC disease includes all cancers with known distant metastases. AJCC staging also contains prefix designations, in which *p* indicates pathologic stage, *c* indicates clinical stage, and *yp* indicates pathologic stage after receiving neoadjuvant treatment (Jessup et al., 2017).

Anal squamous cell staging is clinical in nature and based on clinical examination and diagnostic imaging studies. Tis, or in situ, is reserved for high-grade squamous intraepithelial lesions. T1, T2, and T3 indicate the size of the primary tumor and are 2 cm or less, 2–5 cm, and greater than 5 cm, respectively. T4 is reserved for direct tumor invasion to adjacent organs. Anal cancer lymph node staging is based on location: N1 indicates metastasis in inguinal, mesorectal, internal iliac, or external iliac nodes. N1a signifies metastasis in inguinal, mesorectal, or internal iliac lymph nodes; N1b specifies metastasis in external iliac lymph nodes; and N1c denotes metastasis in external iliac with any N1a nodes (Welton et al., 2017). Stage I is reserved to T1 N0 M0. Stage IIA is T2 N0 M0, whereas stage IIB is T3 N0 M0. Stage IIIA includes T1–2 N1 M0; stage IIIB indicates T4 N0 M0 disease; and stage IIIC denotes T3 N1 M0. Stage IV signifies the presence of any distant metastases, or M1 (Welton et al., 2017).

Treatment

Surgery

In early-stage cT1 or cT2 N0 rectal cancer, transanal excision can be considered in highly selected patients. For localized T3 N0 or greater adenocarcinoma of the colorectum, total mesorectal excision is universally recommended, which includes complete surgical excision with en bloc removal of local lymph nodes, vasculature, and lymphatics. Total mesorectal excision is the only established potentially curative treatment modality for T3 N0 and more advanced colorectal cancer (West et al., 2010). At minimum, 12 regional lymph nodes are needed from a surgical specimen to adequately assess N stage (NCCN, 2018b).

For potentially resectable colon cancer, this may be achieved through either a laparoscopic or open approach. When possible, a laparoscopic approach is associated with reduced perioperative morbidity and mortality and an earlier initiation of adjuvant chemotherapy when indicated (Zheng, Jemal, Lin, Hu, & Chang, 2015).

For potentially resectable rectal cancer, surgical excision should occur after delivery of neoadjuvant therapy with chemoradiation to reduce the risk of local recurrence (Sauer et al., 2004). Transabdominal resection technique varies depending on location. When adequate surgical margins can be achieved with sphincter preservation, low anterior resection is completed. When the tumor location is too low for adequate margins and sphincter preservation, an abdominoperineal resection (APR) is performed, which results in the placement of a permanent colostomy (NCCN, 2018d).

Definitive combination chemotherapy with radiation therapy is the current standard of care in the treatment of anal carcinoma (Czito et al., 2015). Prior to the development of effective chemoradiation, surgical resection with APR was the primary treatment of rectal and anal cancer and was associated with five-year survival of 50%–70% and overall recurrence rate of 40%–60% (Czito et al., 2015). Definitive chemoradiation is associated with improvement in five-year overall survival rates as well as reduced morbidity. However, in patients with persistent or locally recurrent and nonmetastatic disease after completion of chemoradiation, salvage resection with APR remains the standard of care and is associated with five-year survival rates of approximately 50% (Ryan, Compton, & Mayer, 2000).

Preoperative Management

Upfront surgical resection of stage II or III disease is standard practice for potentially resectable cancer of the colon. In contrast, preoperative (neoadjuvant) therapy is the recommended approach in rectal cancer. This recommendation is based on the high local recurrence rates typically seen in rectal cancer not treated with preoperative (neoadjuvant) therapy (Sauer et al., 2004). Current recommendations in management of rectal cancer are for neoadjuvant therapy with a combination of fluoropyrimidine chemotherapy and radiation therapy (NCCN, 2018d). An acceptable alternative is preoperative chemotherapy followed by chemoradiation. The delivery of radiation to the pelvis in conjunction with fluoropyrimidine chemotherapy in the preoperative setting has demonstrated improved rates of local recurrence (6% vs. 13%) and higher rates of sphincter-preserving surgery as compared to chemoradiation given postoperatively (39% vs. 19% sphincter preservation) (Sauer et al., 2004).

Preoperative nursing care involves assessment of patient history and comorbidities, particularly those that may affect patients' ability to successfully recover from surgery. These include personal or family history of myocardial infarction, stroke, chronic kidney disease, diabetes, or other cardiovascular risk factors. Additionally, nurses may screen for history of pulmonary disease and encourage smoking cessation. Assessment of hematologic status is also indicated, and patients with anemia secondary to blood loss from a direct effect of colorectal cancer may require iron replacement or transfusion. Patients who received neoadjuvant treatment should also be screened for recovery of absolute neutrophil count to $1,500/mm^3$ or greater, which is needed for infection prevention, and platelet count of at least $50,000/mm^3$, which is needed to achieve postoperative hemostasis (Lester, 2018).

Postoperative Management

Postoperative care of patients with colorectal cancer requires an interprofessional approach. Nursing care includes assessment of airway, surgical site, and sensorium; pain and nausea management; nutrition support; and monitoring for postoperative complications, including thromboembolism, infection, ileus, and urinary retention. Patient assessment and monitoring of renal function, intake and output, and vital signs are priorities in the immediate postoperative setting (Lester, 2018).

The average length of stay for patients undergoing surgical resection of colorectal cancer is less than five days (Wilkes, 2018). During this window, nurses provide significant patient education. In patients who require an ostomy, a wound and ostomy nurse can provide assessment and individual education. Nurses have a vital role in not only direct patient care, but also patient education. Nurses educate patients regarding reportable symptoms such as fever, shortness of breath, dehiscence, or obstruction. By providing education regarding normal and abnormal symptoms, nurses empower patients to participate in recovery and identify potential complications after discharge. An important component of this education is care coordination, as well as discharge planning and review of the hospital follow-up plan (Wilkes, 2018).

Postoperative (adjuvant) chemotherapy recommendations for localized, completely resected colon cancer vary depending on pathologic stage. Adjuvant chemotherapy is not recommended in patients with stage I or microsatellite instability (MSI)-high (MSI-H) stage II colon cancer (NCCN, 2018b). MSI-H, or deficient mismatch repair (dMMR), colorectal cancer is associated with an overall more favorable prognosis and, in stage II disease, is also associated with lack of benefit from adjuvant chemotherapy (Popat, Hubner, & Houlston, 2005). See High-Risk Assessment: Screening and Genetic Testing for further discussion on MSI.

In patients with low-risk stage II colon cancer, adjuvant chemotherapy with a fluoropyrimidine (either capecitabine or 5-fluorouracil [5-FU]) alone may be considered, but observation is also an appropriate option (NCCN, 2018b). In high-risk stage II colon cancer (T4, poorly differentiated histology, lymphovascular or perineural invasion) and stage III colon cancer, adjuvant chemotherapy with a fluoropyrimidine with or without oxaliplatin can be offered. These recommendations are largely based on the large phase 3 MOSAIC (Multicenter International Study of Oxaliplatin/5-Fluorouracil/Leucovorin in the Adjuvant Treatment of Colon Cancer) study, in which patients with stage II and III colon cancer were randomized to receive six months of adjuvant chemotherapy with 5-FU alone or 5-FU with oxaliplatin (FOLFOX). The study showed an advantage in five-year disease-free survival (DFS) of 73.3% in the FOLFOX group versus 67.4% in the 5-FU group (André et al., 2009). However, this advantage is isolated primarily in patients with lymph node–positive (stage III) resected colon cancer. Patients with stage III colon cancer experienced a higher six-year overall survival of 72.9% in the FOLFOX group, compared with 68.7% in those receiving a fluoropyrimidine alone. This pattern was not seen in a stage II subgroup analysis (André et al., 2009). Adjuvant chemotherapy with a fluoropyrimidine with or without oxaliplatin is also recommended in all patients with clinical stage II or III rectal cancer following neoadjuvant chemoradiation and surgery (NCCN, 2018d). Adjuvant chemotherapy should be initiated as soon as possible because delays in initiation of adjuvant chemotherapy are associated with reductions in survival (Biagi et al., 2011).

Treatment of Metastatic Disease

Colorectal cancer is metastatic at the time of diagnosis in 21% of cases (Siegel et al., 2018). Up to half of patients will develop metastatic disease at some time during the course of the disease (Kanas et al., 2012). Although most cases of metastatic disease are ultimately incurable, resection of metastases has been associated with improvement in overall survival and DFS in patients with resectable metastatic disease to the liver.

In patients with potentially resectable colorectal metastases to the liver, consideration for surgical resection is recommended in patients who are candidates when complete resection is deemed technically feasible. With chemotherapy alone, five-year survival is approximately 10% (Pietrantonio, Garassino, Torri, & Braud, 2012). In oligometastatic liver-only metastatic disease, surgical resection of hepatic metastases is associated with 5- and 10-year survival rates of 25%–40% and 10%–21%, respectively (Abbas, Lam, & Hollands, 2011). Although less common, resection of oligometastatic disease to the lungs is also possible and is associated with improvements in survival (Shah et al., 2006).

A variety of locoregional therapies are available for the treatment of patients with oligometastatic disease that is not resectable because of tumor location. These include external beam radiation, hepatic arterial infusion, radioembolization (radiation-emitting microspheres), transcatheter arterial chemoembolization with drug-eluding beads, tumor ablation with radiofrequency ablation, cryoablation, microwave ablation, and percutaneous ethanol ablation. Although radiofrequency ablation is the most studied, similar response rates have been found across the aforementioned modalities (Zacharias et al., 2015).

In combination with chemotherapy, liver-directed treatment with radiofrequency ablation to liver metastases has been shown to offer improvements in progression-free and overall survival as compared with chemotherapy alone in patients with liver-only unresectable disease that is amenable to liver-directed therapies (Ruers et al., 2017).

Surgical resection and liver-directed therapies are reserved for cases of stage IV disease that are completely addressed by resection or ablative approaches, and resection is not performed in cases in which all known sites of disease cannot be treated with appropriate margins (NCCN, 2018b). Chemotherapy and locoregional approaches can be used with a goal of conversion to resectability (NCCN, 2018b). In cases of unresectable metastatic disease, supportive care with or without chemotherapy is integral, with the goal of improving quality of life and life expectancy.

Metastatic anal squamous cell cancer is relatively rare, occurring in approximately 5% of cases at the time of diagnosis and another 20% of cases after primary treatment (Eng et al., 2014). Because of the rarity of the diagnosis, large randomized studies evaluating systemic therapies are lacking. The most studied combination is 5-FU with cisplatin, which remains the standard first-line regimen in the treatment of metastatic anal cancer.

Chemotherapy

Chemotherapy agents used in the perioperative setting in the care of patients with colorectal cancer include fluoropyrimidines with or without oxaliplatin. These agents are also approved in the management of metastatic disease. Other agents approved in the metastatic setting include irinotecan and, in refractory disease, trifluridine-tipiracil.

Nursing care includes assessment of and nursing intervention for toxicities of therapy (see Table 1-2). Mucositis is commonly experienced in fluoropyrimidine-containing regimens, and prophylaxis with oral hygiene and an oral care protocol is recommended (Jackson, Johnson, Sosman, Murphy, & Epstein, 2015). Diarrhea is commonly experienced by patients treated with fluoropyrimidine- and irinotecan-containing regimens and can have a significant impact on quality of life, as well as lead to disturbances in fluid and electrolyte balance. Aggressive antidiarrheal management with oral loperamide is recommended, as well as injectable octreotide for refractory diarrhea (Stern & Ippoliti, 2003).

Palmar-plantar erythrodysesthesia, also known as hand-foot syndrome, is a common adverse effect of fluoropyrimidine-containing regimens (Nagore, Insa, & Sanmartin, 2000). Symptoms include erythema, edema, pain, and, in severe cases, blistering and desquamation. When applied regularly, 10% urea cream has shown clinical benefit in prevention of palmar-plantar erythrodysesthesia (Hofheinz et al., 2015).

Oxaliplatin is associated with neuropathic symptoms, both acute and chronic. Reactions that commonly occur during or immediately after infusion include cold-induced dysesthesia, dyspnea, muscle cramps, jaw stiffness, fasciculations, and voice and ocular changes (Pachman et al., 2015). Patient education regarding cold avoidance is indicated, and decreasing the rate of infusion may be considered. Persistent peripheral neuropathy also can develop, with incidence and intensity increasing with cumulative exposure. Patients receiving oxaliplatin should be

Table 1-2. Chemotherapy for Colorectal Cancer

Agent	Indications	Common Toxicities
Fluoropyrimidines (including 5-FU and capecitabine)	Adjuvant, monotherapy, in combination with radiation; metastatic, in combination with oxaliplatin or irinotecan	Fatigue, palmar-plantar erythrodysesthesia, diarrhea, stomatitis/mucositis, anemia, neutropenia, thrombocytopenia
Irinotecan	Metastatic, as monotherapy or in combination with 5-FU	Cholinergic syndrome (diaphoresis, flushing, increased peristalsis, lacrimation, miosis, rhinitis, sialorrhea), alopecia, diarrhea, nausea, abdominal pain, abdominal cramping, vomiting, anemia, neutropenia, thrombocytopenia, increased bilirubin
Oxaliplatin	Adjuvant, in combination with fluoropyrimidine; metastatic, in combination with fluoropyrimidine	Fatigue, acute neuropathy, chronic neuropathy, paresthesia, neutropenia, thrombocytopenia, anemia, nausea, allergic reaction
Trifluridine-tipiracil	Metastatic, after progression on fluoropyrimidine, oxaliplatin, irinotecan, and agents targeted against VEGF and EGFR (in *RAS* wild type)	Neutropenia, anemia, thrombocytopenia, fatigue, asthenia

EGFR—epidermal growth factor receptor; 5-FU—5-fluorouracil; VEGF—vascular endothelial growth factor

Note. Based on information from André et al., 2004; Cassidy et al., 2008; Mayer et al., 2015; Pfizer Inc., 2016.

routinely assessed for the presence or worsening of persistent numbness or paresthesias. Patients on oxaliplatin often require dose reduction or permanent discontinuation, especially when pain, motor weakness, or interference with instrumental activities of daily living is present (Hershman, Lacchetti, & Loprinzi, 2014).

Definitive combination chemoradiation is the standard of care in the treatment of nonmetastatic squamous cell carcinoma of the anus. The chemotherapeutic component of therapy includes 5-FU 1,000 mg/m^2/day on days 1–4 and 29–32 and mitomycin C 10 mg/m^2 on days 1 and 29 (Flam et al., 1996). Colostomy-free survival and DFS with this approach were 71% and 73%, respectively, in a large randomized phase 3 study (Flam et al., 1996). Alternatively, capecitabine may be administered at a dose of 825 mg/m² twice a day on days of radiation along with mitomycin C (Glynne-Jones et al., 2008). Toxicities frequently related to these regimens include fluoropyrimidine-associated toxicity as discussed previously and in Table 1-2. Additional toxicities include high-grade cytopenias and neutropenia, which are related to the addition of mitomycin C. Nursing care includes monitoring and intervention for signs and symptoms of anemia, thrombocytopenia, and neutropenia, as well as supportive measures for perianal discomfort related to both the tumor effect and radiation effect (see Radiation Therapy).

Targeted Therapy

Active targeted therapies in the management of metastatic disease include agents targeting vascular endothelial growth factor (VEGF) and epidermal growth factor receptor (EGFR). Agents targeting VEGF include bevacizumab, ziv-aflibercept, ramucirumab, and, in refractory disease, regorafenib.

The management of metastatic colorectal cancer is biomarker driven. Molecular testing for mutations in the biomarkers *NRAS* and *KRAS* is standard, and mutations in these genes confer resistance to agents targeting EGFR (Allegra, Rumble, & Schilsky, 2016). The anti-EGFR monoclonal antibodies cetuximab and panitumumab are approved in the setting of metastatic colorectal cancer without mutations in *NRAS* or *KRAS* (with *RAS* wild-type disease).

An important nursing consideration in the care of patients receiving targeted therapies is monitoring for the specific toxicities associated with these agents and implementing management strategies. In patients treated with VEGF-targeted agents, blood pressure and urine protein monitoring is indicated. Anti-EGFR monoclonal antibodies are associated with treatment-related acneform eruption. Reducing sun exposure through the use of protective clothing or sunblock, application of moisturizing lotion, and prophylactic therapy with oral doxycycline and topical hydrocortisone cream has proved effective in reducing rash severity (Lacouture et al., 2010).

To date, no targeted therapies have been approved in the treatment of anal squamous cell cancer. The anti-EGFR monoclonal antibody cetuximab, which has demonstrated activity in other HPV-related cancers, was investigated in combination with standard chemoradiation. Unfortunately, the investigation was discontinued because of unacceptable toxicity observed in the patients receiving standard therapy plus cetuximab (Deutsch et al., 2013).

Immunotherapy

The development of cancer involves a multistep process. One component of oncogenesis is the evasion of cancer cells from normal, appropriate immune response, which is destruction of malignant and premalignant cells (Vinay et al., 2015). Complex signaling between human T cells and antigen-presenting cells occurs during normal immune surveillance. Programmed cell death protein 1 (PD-1) is an inhibitory molecule located on T lymphocytes. Anti-PD-1 monoclonal antibodies act by blocking immune inhibition. These agents have shown activity in a molecular subset of MSI-H metastatic colorectal cancer (Le et al., 2015).

The anti-PD-1 monoclonal antibodies pembrolizumab and nivolumab are indicated in the setting of metastatic MSI-H colorectal cancer that has progressed on chemotherapy (Le et al., 2016; Overman et al., 2017). Clinical benefit was shown for pembrolizumab in heavily pretreated MSI-H metastatic colon cancer in the form of a 50% objective response rate and an 89% disease control rate, defined as objective response or stable disease at six-month follow-up (Le et al., 2016). Nivolumab showed similar activity in heavily pretreated MSI-H metastatic colon cancer with an objective response rate of 31% and a disease control rate of 61% (Overman et al., 2017).

The activity of anti-PD-1 therapy has also been demonstrated in metastatic anal squamous cell carcinoma. One factor in the oncogenesis of chronic HPV infection is upregulation of immune checkpoint proteins, including PD-1. Nivolumab demonstrated a response rate of 24%, including two patients with complete response, in a small, single-arm study in patients with chemorefractory, metastatic anal squamous cell carcinoma (Morris et al., 2017).

The PD-1 monoclonal antibodies are associated with a unique, immune-associated toxicity profile. Nurses should assess for the presence of immune-related toxicities associated with anti-PD-1 antibodies. These include generalized symptoms such as fatigue and rash. Immune-mediated colitis has been identified, ranging from diarrhea to hematochezia. Autoimmune thyroiditis also can occur, manifested as alterations in thyroid-stimulating hormone, which is routinely monitored. Less commonly, autoimmune pneumonitis, hypophysitis, pancreatitis, arthritis, hepatitis, and nephritis have been identified. Interventions for immune-mediated toxicity vary depending on severity but include holding therapy and administering corticosteroids (Naidoo et al., 2015).

See Table 1-3 for a listing of targeted and immunotherapy agents used in the treatment of colorectal cancer, as well as their common toxicities.

Radiation Therapy

Radiation therapy is indicated in several applications in the treatment of colon, rectal, and anal carcinomas. Neoadjuvant chemoradiation is the standard approach in the treatment of potentially resectable

Table 1-3. Targeted and Immunotherapy Agents for Colorectal Cancer

Agent/Class	Indication	Common Toxicities
Anti-EGFR monoclonal antibodies: cetuximab and panitumumab	KRAS and NRAS wild-type metastatic colorectal cancer	Acneform rash, conjunctivitis, diarrhea, hypomagnesemia, paronychia
Anti-PD-1 monoclonal antibodies: pembrolizumab and nivolumab	MSI-H metastatic colorectal cancer	Colitis, diarrhea/endocrinopathy, fatigue, immune-mediated thyroid dysregulation, increase in alanine aminotransferase, rash
Anti-VEGF monoclonal antibodies: bevacizumab, regorafenib, ziv-aflibercept	Metastatic colorectal cancer, in combination with fluoropyrimidine-based chemotherapy	Bleeding, delayed wound healing, hypertension, proteinuria, thromboembolism
Regorafenib	Metastatic colorectal cancer, after progression on fluoropyrimidine, oxaliplatin, irinotecan, bevacizumab, and if RAS wild type	Diarrhea, hand-foot skin reaction, fatigue, hypertension, rash or desquamation

EGFR—epidermal growth factor receptor; MSI-H—microsatellite instability high; PD-1—programmed cell death protein 1; VEGF—vascular endothelial growth factor

Note. Based on information from Genentech, Inc., 2018; Grothey et al., 2013; Le et al., 2015; Naidoo et al., 2015; Van Cutsem et al., 2009.

T3–T4 and lymph node–positive rectal cancer (NCCN, 2018d). This approach has been shown to reduce local recurrence rates and result in higher rates of sphincter-preserving surgery compared to upfront surgery (Sauer et al., 2004). Palliative radiation therapy also is indicated in the treatment of symptomatic metastatic lesions. Definitive chemoradiation with 5-FU and mitomycin C is the standard-of-care treatment for anal squamous cell carcinoma (Flam et al., 1996).

Nursing assessment for radiation-related toxicities includes monitoring for signs and symptoms of radiation dermatitis. These include discomfort, erythema, dry desquamation, and moist desquamation. For erythema or dry desquamation, 0.2% hyaluronic acid cream and calendula cream may be of benefit, although studies showing benefit were not performed in patients receiving radiation therapy for rectal cancer. For moist desquamation, dressings are recommended, and antimicrobial therapy should be considered if wound cultures demonstrate infection (Feight, Baney, Bruce, & McQuestion, 2011).

Radiation therapy to the pelvis also is associated with infertility risk. Patients should be counseled regarding these risks and offered referral to a fertility preservation specialist for consideration of sperm, oocyte, or ovarian tissue banking. Additionally, radiation therapy to the pelvis may cause vaginal stenosis. The use of a vaginal dilator is recommended following completion of radiation therapy, but not during (Morris, Do, Chard, & Brand, 2017).

Radiation-induced colitis results from radiation-induced stem cell damage to colonic epithelium. Symptoms include diarrhea, nausea, vomiting, anorexia, and pain. Supportive treatment directed at controlling symptoms is indicated, including antidiarrheal management with loperamide or octreotide, and analgesia (Zimmerer, Böcker, Wenz, & Singer, 2008).

Guidelines for Treatment

NCCN guidelines summarize expert recommendations for the management of various cancers. Surgical resection followed by consideration of adjuvant chemotherapy, as summarized in the preceding sections, is the NCCN recommendation for stage II and III colorectal adenocarcinoma (NCCN, 2018b). Similarly, NCCN outlines recommendations for neoadjuvant chemoradiation followed by surgical resection in stage T3 N0 or greater rectal cancer, as detailed previously (NCCN, 2018d).

NCCN guidelines for the management of stage IV colon and rectal cancer include the recommendation for surgical consideration for metastasectomy for liver and lung metastases and consideration of liver-directed therapies only in patients with disease that can be completely addressed by directed approaches (NCCN, 2018b, 2018d). Chemotherapy, targeted therapy, and immunotherapy options are listed in detail, as have been summarized earlier in this chapter.

Finally, NCCN guidelines for the management of anal cancer advocate for definitive chemoradiation with a fluoropyrimidine and mitomycin C, as described previously (NCCN, 2018a). Additionally, NCCN guidelines for colon, rectal, and anal cancer describe consensus recommendations for survivorship and surveillance (see Surveillance and Survivorship).

Clinical Trials Influencing Current Treatment

The current standard duration of adjuvant chemotherapy after resection of stage III colon cancer is six months. The persistent neurotoxicity associated with oxaliplatin represents a significant quality-of-life issue in colorectal cancer survivors treated with oxaliplatin. This is related to cumulative dose and was persistent at four years for more than 13% of patients treated with six months of oxaliplatin in the adjuvant setting enrolled in the MOSAIC study (André et al., 2009). Given these findings, six collaborating clinical trials are currently investigating the comparison of three months' duration of adjuvant chemotherapy with 5-FU and oxaliplatin versus six months' duration (Shi et al., 2017). If found noninferior, three months of adjuvant therapy may become a new standard, which could potentially result in a considerable reduction in neuropathic morbidity, but more mature data are needed before these findings can be applied to standard practice.

The current standard in the management of locally advanced rectal cancer involves neoadjuvant chemoradiation followed by surgical resection (see Preoperative Management). The rates of pathologic complete response of approximately 25% raise the clinical question as to whether surgical resection is required in patients with a complete response to chemoradiation. An ongoing area of investigation involves the watch-and-wait approach to follow-up, which offers the potential for patients who have a complete pathologic response to avoid the morbidity associated with surgery (Plummer, Leake, & Albert, 2017). Challenges to this approach include the lack of criteria for determining complete pathologic response, and NCCN (2018d) does not advocate for this practice outside of clinical trials.

Recent approvals in immunotherapy with the anti-PD-1 monoclonal antibodies pembrolizumab and nivolumab in the treatment of MSI-H/dMMR metastatic refractory colorectal cancer are based on interim analysis at 6 and 12 months, respectively, of ongoing clinical trials showing significant benefit, leading to accelerated approvals. Long-term follow-up is ongoing, as these trials remain open at the time of this publication (Le et al., 2016; Overman et al., 2017).

Although these breakthroughs in immunotherapy are promising, current benefit from anti-PD-1 therapies in colorectal cancer is restricted to patients with MSI-H/dMMR tumors, which represent 10%–20% of all cases of colorectal cancer but only 3.5%–5% of the total number of patients with metastatic colorectal cancer (Koopman et al., 2009). An important focus for future investigation is expanding the utility of immunotherapy approaches in microsatellite stable (MSS) metastatic colon cancer. One ongoing trial is investigating the combination of atezolizumab, an anti–programmed cell death-ligand 1 antibody, with cobimetinib, an MEK inhibitor, to increase immune destruction of cancer cells. Preliminary data confirmed responses in a small number of patients, including patients with MSS disease (Bendell et al., 2016).

Nursing Care

The care of patients with colorectal and anal cancer involves assessment and intervention for symptoms related to both the cancer and side effects from therapy. Nurses have an invaluable role in the safe administration of chemotherapy that encompasses verification of dosing accuracy, assessment of contraindications and toxicities, patient education regarding reportable side effects, and symptom management (Wilkes, 2018). Prior to administration of chemotherapy, the oncology nurse assessment includes review of laboratory results to ensure that appropriate hematologic, renal, and hepatic parameters are met. Nurses also perform the key role of ensuring safe and appropriate administration of chemotherapy and immunotherapy. Oncology nurses monitor for acute and delayed toxicities throughout and after administration. Knowledge of toxicities specific to given therapies is critical to appropriately assess patient tolerance and outcomes (see Chemotherapy, Targeted Therapy, and Immunotherapy). Chemotherapy side effects can be severe and even life threatening, and oncology nurses are critical in promoting patient safety and positive outcomes through assessment, education, and implementation of nursing interventions (Wilkes, 2018).

Oncology nurses also perform a critical role in interprofessional management of symptoms secondary to colorectal cancer. Bowel obstruction is a complication of colorectal cancer that can result from internal or external compression by tumor on the bowel, leading to blockage. This can present as pain, nausea, vomiting, reduction or absence of bowel movements, and reduced bowel sounds on physical assessment. If obstruction is suspected, abdominal x-ray or CT can be used for identification and is aided by ingestion of oral contrast (Wilkes, 2018). The management of obstruction includes gut rest with placement of a nasogastric tube for decompression and administration of IV fluids. Surgical consultation is indicated to evaluate the possibility of surgical intervention to relieve obstruction. Additional management includes pharmacotherapy to palliate pain, nausea, and vomiting (Wilkes, 2018).

Symptoms related to colorectal cancer can result from direct mass effect of the primary or metastatic tumors. The liver is the most common site of metastases, and the presence of metastatic lesions within the liver can progress to liver failure. This presents as jaundice, nausea, anorexia, edema, hypoalbuminemia, ascites, and altered mentation. Peritoneal involvement can also lead to the development of ascites. From either cause, ascites can cause shortness of breath, pain, and early satiety. Interventions to address ascites include paracentesis, diuretic administration, and nutrition interventions to improve serum albumin (Wilkes, 2018). An additional symptom experienced is anorexia-cachexia syndrome. Small, frequent meals and antiemetic administration are recommended. Total parenteral nutrition is not recommended unless aggressive treatment can result in reversing the disease state (Wilkes, 2018). Patients with advanced disease causing visceral pain often require opioid analgesia for palliation. Assessing for and preventing constipation through an appropriate bowel regimen is a critical nursing intervention, as constipation can result from opioid analgesia and exacerbate abdominal pain symptoms (Wilkes, 2018).

Throughout the continuum of care, oncology nurses are tasked with critical roles in the assessment and management of patients with colorectal and anal cancer.

Prognosis

The five-year overall survival rate for colorectal cancer for all stages combined is 65% (Siegel et al., 2018). The five-year survival rates for localized, regional, and distant stages at diagnosis are 90%, 71%, and 14%, respectively (Siegel et al., 2018).

In rectal cancer treated with neoadjuvant chemoradiation, degree of treatment response is highly prognostic. This was demonstrated by long-term data from the CAO/ARO/AIO-94 trial, showing that patients with the greatest degree of tumor regression had a 10-year DFS of 90%, whereas those with no tumor regression had a 10-year DFS of 63% (Fokas et al., 2014).

MSI-H status refers to alterations in mismatch repair genes associated with repeated sequences called microsatellites. *Microsatellite stable, or MSS,* refers to tumors with intact mismatch repair genes. MSI is a useful marker in screening for hereditary nonpolyposis colorectal cancer (see High-Risk Assessment: Screening and Genetic Testing) and is predictive of potential benefit from anti-PD-1 antibodies. In addition, in stage II and III colorectal cancer, MSI-H is a useful prognostic indicator. The six-year survival rates for MSI-H versus MSS resected stage II colorectal cancer are 97% and 82%, respectively. Similarly, the six-year survival rates for stage III resected colorectal cancer are 78% in MSI-H and 56% in MSS (Lanza et al., 2006).

Additional pathologic prognostic indicators can be gathered from pathologic features, with positive surgical margins, lymphovascular or perineural invasion, and poorly differentiated histology, as discussed previously (see Histology).

The prognosis for anal squamous cell carcinoma is relatively good with definitive chemoradiation, with reported DFS of 73%–80% after completion of treatment with combination radiation therapy and fluoropyrimidine plus mitomycin C chemotherapy (Bartelink et al., 1997; Flam et al., 1996). Despite relatively good outcomes overall, retrospective review of the large RTOG 98-11 trial demonstrated that higher-risk features are associated with less favorable prognosis. T stage is a significant prognostic indicator; T2 stage is associated with 82% overall survival, whereas patients with T4 lymph node–negative disease had 57% overall survival. Lymph node–positive disease is also associated with reduced overall survival of 42%–57% (Gunderson et al., 2013). In addition, skin ulceration and male sex are also associated with poorer prognosis overall (Bartelink et al., 1997).

Prevention

Screening colonoscopy allows for the direct visualization and removal of precancerous polyps and early-stage cancers. An estimated 73%–91% of colorectal cancer is preventable by screening colonoscopy (Brenner et al., 2007). Although colorectal adenocarcinoma rates are trending downward overall in the United States, colonoscopic screening remains underutilized. Unfortunately, up to 90% of colorectal adenocarcinoma continues to be diagnosed in the more advanced, symptomatic stage (Moreno et al., 2016).

A number of lifestyle factors have been associated with reduced risk for developing colorectal cancer. A systematic review and meta-analysis demonstrated that the most physically active people have an approximately 25% reduced risk for developing colorectal cancer as compared with the least physically active (Boyle, Keegel, Bull, Heyworth, & Fritschi, 2012). Epidemiologic evidence supports the association between diet and colorectal cancer. Vegetarian, pescatarian, and semi-vegetarian diets were associated with lower risk of colorectal cancer. In the large, prospective Adventist Health Study-2, the respective hazard ratios for development in these groups were 0.82, 0.57, and 0.92, compared with matched nonvegetarians (Orlich et al., 2015). Diets high in fiber are also associated with a reduced risk of developing colorectal cancer (Aune et al., 2011).

Regular aspirin use has also been associated with reduced risk of colorectal cancer. A systematic review and meta-analysis demonstrated significantly reduced rates of colon and rectal cancer in individuals who took aspirin 75 mg or more daily (Rothwell et al., 2010). The U.S. Preventive Services Task Force recommends low-dose daily aspirin in people aged 50–59 on the basis of established chemoprotective effect, citing both cardiovascular and colorectal cancer outcomes (Bibbins-Domingo, 2016). Aspirin use may also have value in secondary prevention in patients diagnosed with colorectal cancer and has been demonstrated to be associated with improved disease-specific and overall survival in this population (Bains et al., 2016).

The majority of anal squamous cell cancers result from chronic infection with oncogenic HPV type 16 (Daling et al., 2004). Anal intercourse is associated with the development of HPV-related dysplastic cytology and anal HPV infection (Moscicki et al., 1999). A sequence of progression from low-grade to high-grade neoplasia has been identified, and high-grade, p16-positive anal intraepithelial neoplasia is considered a premalignant condition analogous to neoplasia identified in cervical specimens. Given the biologic similarity with cervical cancer (HPV related, squamous histology), screening for anal intraepithelial neoplasia in a similar fashion in at-risk populations has been proposed, with sensitivity and specificity comparable to that seen in cervical cancer screening (Czito et al., 2015). At this time, data from large, randomized trials supporting cytologic screening are lacking, and further study is needed before large-scale cytological screening programs can be instituted (Chiao, Giordano, Palefsky, Tyring, & Serag, 2006).

Vaccination against HPV types 6, 11, 16, and 18 has demonstrated effectiveness in the prevention of infection with these strains of HPV and the development of genital warts (Giuliano et al., 2011). Furthermore, a study in a high-risk population demonstrated immunization with vaccination against HPV types 6, 11, 16, and 18 to be associated with a 78% reduction in the development of high-grade anal intraepithelial neoplasia and an 84% reduction in the detection of HPV DNA (Palefsky et al., 2011). This supports the hypothesis that HPV vaccination has the potential to prevent anal carcinoma through prevention of chronic HPV infection, which is the most common etiology for the development of anal carcinoma.

High-Risk Assessment: Screening and Genetic Testing

Although the majority of colorectal cancer cases are sporadic in nature, a number of inheritable familial syndromes are known (see Table 1-1). Of these, Lynch syndrome is the most common, accounting for approximately 2%–4% of all cases of colorectal cancer (Lynch & Chapelle, 2003). Lynch syndrome is an autosomal dominant disorder that results from inherited mutation in one of four DNA MMR genes: *MLH1*, *MSH2*, *MSH6*, and *PMS2* (Palomaki, McClain, Melillo, Hampel, & Thibodeau, 2009). These genes code for DNA MMR proteins, which normally correct errors in DNA replication occurring during cellular division.

Alteration in MMR genes results in increased accumulation of redundant genetic nucleotide mismatch mutations known as *microsatellite instability,* or *MSI* (Hendriks et al., 2006). Accumulation of increased mutations in cancer-related genes leads to an increased rate of oncogenesis (Lynch & Chapelle, 2003). Tumor specimens can be tested for expression of MMR proteins or MSI. Although both methodologies share high sensitivity and specificity, MSI testing has a disadvantage in that it does not provide insight into which gene or protein is implicated (Hendriks et al., 2006).

It is important to identify Lynch syndrome in patients and families because of the high rates of second Lynch syndrome–associated primary cancers in the same individual and its dominant inheritance pattern, which is commonly passed on to first-degree relatives. Lynch syndrome–associated colorectal cancers typically develop at a younger age and are more likely to be right sided (Lynch & Chapelle, 2003). In individuals with Lynch syndrome, the lifetime risk for developing colorectal cancer varies from 12% to 48% depending on the genes involved (Bonadona et al., 2011). Lynch syndrome is also associated with an increased risk for the development of multiple extracolonic cancers, including endometrial, gastric, small bowel, urothelial, brain (glioma), and ovarian cancer (Lynch & Chapelle, 2003).

NCCN (2018c) recommends universal screening of all colorectal cancer specimens for Lynch syndrome–associated molecular profile. This screening can be completed with one of two methodologies: (a) immunohistochemistry analysis for MMR protein (*MLH1*, *MSH2*, *MSH6*, and *PMS2*) expression, or (b) analysis for MSI, a result of MMR protein deficiency. More than 90% of Lynch syndrome specimens are MSI-H and lack normal expression of one of the four MMR proteins. Abnormal initial screening results must be interpreted in clinical context, as 10%–15% of sporadic, nonfamilial colorectal cancers also express this molecular profile (French et al., 2008). Sporadic MSI-H colorectal cancer is associated with hypermethylation of *MLH1*, a feature that can be identified by the presence of *BRAF* mutation, which rules out Lynch syndrome in MSI-H colorectal cancers (Deng et al., 2004). In addition to molecular markers, clinical criteria exist to identify individuals at risk for Lynch syndrome. The Amsterdam II criteria identify at-risk individuals as having the following: (a) three relatives with a Lynch syndrome–associated cancer, one of which is a first-degree relative of the other two, (b) two successive generations affected, and (c) at least one case being diagnosed before age 50. In addition, familial adenomatous polyposis should be excluded (Vasen, Watson, Mecklin, & Lynch, 1999). When clinical concern for Lynch syndrome is present on the basis of clinical context and MSI-H or abnormality in MMR proteins, germline testing may be conducted to differentiate sporadic MSI-H cancers from Lynch syndrome. This should be performed in consultation with a genetics expert (NCCN, 2018c).

If a deleterious germline mutation is identified, institution of Lynch syndrome surveillance is indicated. This includes surveillance for colon cancer, endometrial and ovarian cancer, and less frequently associated cancers, including gastric, small bowel, and urothelial cancers. Screening colonoscopy every one to two years starting at age 20–25 is recommended because of the relatively rapid progression from polyp to cancer seen in Lynch syndrome (Lynch & Chapelle, 2003). Although no active surveillance for endometrial or ovarian cancer is established in this population, patient education regarding reportable signs and symptoms, such as dysfunctional uterine bleeding, is advised. Prophylactic total abdominal hysterectomy with bilateral salpingo-oophorectomy is an option in women who have completed childbearing (Schmeler et al., 2006). Urinalysis is also recommended annually for screening of urothelial cancers (Mork et al., 2015). In addition to screening of the affected individual, screening of at-risk family members is indicated. This includes first-degree relatives, as well as more distant family members if first-degree relatives are unwilling or unable to be tested (NCCN, 2018c). Finally, chemoprevention with aspirin is associated with reduction in cancer incidence in carriers of Lynch hereditary colon cancer genes (Burn et al., 2011).

Surveillance

After curative intent therapy is complete, consensus recommendations are for disease surveillance (Meyerhardt et al., 2013). The goals of surveillance are to identify recurrences that may be amenable to cure, identify new primary colorectal neoplasms before they become invasive, and monitor for delayed complications of therapies received. In all stages treated with curative intent, endoscopic surveillance one year from resection is indicated, with subsequent endoscopy at three- and five-year intervals afterward. When premalignant polyps are identified, annual endoscopic surveillance is recommended until the patient is polyp free. Serial CEA monitoring is also recommended and has been shown, when applying a threshold of 5 mcg/L, to provide sensitivity of 71% and specificity of 88% in identification of recurrent disease (Nicholson et al., 2015). Although CEA testing is helpful, the sensitivity of CEA monitoring with the goal of early identification of potentially curable recurrences is below the acceptable threshold to function as a stand-alone approach to surveillance (Nicholson et al., 2015). Thus, in patients with a history of stage II and III colorectal cancer, strategies incorporating both CEA testing and advanced imaging of the chest, abdomen, and pelvis with CT are recommended, in addition to history and physical examination, serum chemistries including liver function panel, and complete blood count (NCCN, 2018b).

The approach of more intensive surveillance has been demonstrated to identify a significant number of patients with potentially resectable metastatic recurrences. When identified, these patients then receive definitive therapy for the recurrences with the goal of achieving remission, with 30% of patients identified as having liver-only metastases during surveillance imaging achieving remission at five-year follow-up (Primrose et al., 2014).

The frequency of recommended monitoring is based on recurrence patterns. In a pooled analysis of 20,898 survivors of stage II and III colorectal cancer, 80% of recurrences were identified to have occurred within three years of surgery, and 8% occurred between years 3 and 5 (Sargent et al., 2005). Thus, intensive surveillance with CEA monitoring and CT imaging is advised every three to six months for two years, then every 6–12 months for five years (NCCN, 2018b).

Surveillance after primary treatment of anal cancer with definitive chemoradiation involves monitoring for local response or treatment failure and periodic monitoring for metastatic disease. Digital rectal examination and inguinal lymph node palpation should occur 8–12 weeks after completion of chemoradiation to assess for response. If a complete clinical response has occurred at 8–12 weeks, this examination is repeated every 3–6 months for 5 years (NCCN, 2018a). If biopsy-proven residual disease is present at the time of the first follow-up, the determination regarding salvage surgery with APR versus close observation is based on whether evidence of progressive disease is present (NCCN, 2018a). This recommendation is based on findings that 72% of patients who had residual disease on examination at 11 weeks after chemoradiation went on to show a complete response by 26 months (James et al., 2013). If persistent residual disease, progressive local disease, or local recurrence is identified, surgical resection with APR is recommended, which has resulted in a 50% five-year DFS (Czito et al., 2015). Additional surveillance recommendations include anoscopy every 6–12 months for five years, and chest, abdomen, and pelvis CT imaging with contrast yearly for three years (NCCN, 2018a).

Survivorship

Upon completion of primary treatment of cancer, the focus of cancer care shifts to survivorship care. Colorectal cancer survivors are the third largest survivorship population, representing 11% of the total survivorship population (Hewitt, Greenfield, & Stovall, 2006). Focused assessment for quality-of-life components is essential in providing quality survivorship care. Colorectal cancer survivors have been identified as having a higher risk for developing depression, indicating a need for distress screening and appropriate intervention (Ramsey, Berry, Moinpour, Giedzinska, & Andersen, 2002). Patients with colorectal cancer may experience chronic bowel pattern changes. Patients may report loose stools or an increase in stool frequency after colonic resection, which tends to improve over time (Hewitt et al., 2006). Adhesions secondary to surgery or radiation therapy can lead to abdominal pain or bowel obstruction. Education regarding measures to improve bowel pattern, such as including fiber and the use of over-the-counter stool softeners, is of benefit (Hewitt et al., 2006).

Rectal cancer survivors may experience sexual dysfunction secondary to injury to pelvic nerves and vasculature from cancer and cancer therapy. Male patients can experience erectile dysfunction, which may require medications or referral to urology. Female patients can experience painful coitus. Interventions include use of a vaginal dilator and over-the-counter lubricants (Vogel, 2017). A significant percentage of patients who received oxaliplatin also experience chronic peripheral neuropathy (Hershman et al., 2014).

Survivorship care includes educating patients and promoting lifestyle modifications known to improve colorectal cancer outcomes and overall health. Lifestyle factors including smoking cessation, maintenance of a healthy body mass index, and regular physical exercise have been identified as beneficial for improving colorectal cancer outcomes. Increased physical activity has been shown to reduce mortality in colorectal cancer survivor populations (Campbell, Patel, Newton, Jacobs, & Gapstur, 2013). Increases in activity by any amount in colorectal cancer survivors have been associated with decreased mortality, with greater improvements shown in patients who engaged in moderate exercise for at least 150 minutes per week (Schmid & Leitzmann, 2014). A diet higher in vegetables and fruit, whole grains, poultry, and fish and lower in refined grains, red and processed meat, and refined sugars is associated with lower recurrence and improved overall survival (Meyerhardt et al., 2007).

Survivorship care in patients treated for anal cancers involves monitoring for late toxicities of pelvic radiation. Anal cancer survivors commonly report global reduction in quality of life, fatigue, dyspnea, insomnia, diarrhea, fecal incontinence, increased stool frequency, buttock pain, flatulence, erectile dysfunction (males), dyspareunia, and reduced sexual interest following therapy with combined chemotherapy and pelvic radiation (Bentzen et al., 2013). Unique screening and prevention elements of survivorship care planning in anal cancer survivors includes considering screening for HIV status. Additionally, cervical screening for female patients is also recommended because of the shared etiology between anal and cervical cancers.

Goals of survivorship care include prevention of new and recurrent cancers, prevention of late effects of cancer and cancer therapy, intervention for consequences of cancer and cancer therapy, and coordination of care between the oncology team and primary care provider to ensure that all healthcare needs are comprehensively met (Hewitt et al., 2006). The Health and Medicine Division of the National Academies of Sciences, Engineering, and Medicine (formerly the Institute of Medicine) and other bodies have promoted written survivorship care plans as a standard of care for facilitating improved outcomes in cancer survivors. The survivorship care plan provides a written summary of the treatment received, possible late side effects of cancer and cancer therapy, information on reportable signs of recurrence, recommendations for follow-up, lifestyle recommendations, and defined roles between the oncology and primary care provider. The plan should be given to the patient and primary care provider (Hewitt et al., 2006).

Survivorship care also includes disease prevention, such as immunizations, screening for second cancers, and routine health care, in collaboration with the primary care team.

Summary

Collectively, cancers of the colon, rectum, and anus represent a significant health burden. Although colon and rectal cancer rates have declined overall, they remain the third most common form of cancer, as well as the third leading cause of cancer death in men and women (Siegel et al., 2018). Additionally, colon and rectal cancer rates are increasing rapidly in people younger than age 50 (Siegel et al., 2017). Despite being a relatively uncommon malignancy, anal cancer rates have more than doubled in recent decades (Nelson et al., 2013).

Evidence-based interprofessional care is needed for the promotion of improved outcomes for patients affected by cancers of the colon, rectum, and anus. Oncology nurses can promote prevention of these cancers by encouraging screening colonoscopy in asymptomatic patients. Nurses may also educate patients on high-risk familial syndromes and provide referral to genetic counseling as indicated. Furthermore, nurses have a role in educating patients regarding the signs and symptoms that indicate evaluation.

Nurses are better suited to provide appropriate patient care and education in the context of understanding disease biology, therapeutic options, and goals of therapy. Nurses can both educate and advocate for patients in the setting of the overall clinical picture. By remaining apprised of the most current therapies, nurses have the opportunity to promote best practice.

Patients with cancers of the colon, rectum, and anus commonly experience significant disease-related symptoms, including pain, fatigue, anorexia, nausea, vomiting, diarrhea, obstruction, and depression. In addition, patients also may experience significant toxicities related to radiation, chemotherapy, and surgery. Oncology nurses have a vital role in assessment for these related symptoms. When symptoms are identified, nurses collaborate with the patient, family, and medical team to develop a plan that includes nursing interventions to address these toxicities. In doing so, nurses have the opportunity to promote improved quality of life and, potentially, disease outcomes.

References

Abbas, S., Lam, V., & Hollands, M. (2011). Ten-year survival after liver resection for colorectal metastases: Systematic review and meta-analysis. *ISRN Oncology, 2011,* 1–11. https://doi.org/10.5402/2011/763245

Ahnen, D.J., Wade, S.W., Jones, W.F., Sifri, R., Silveiras, J.M., Greenamyer, J., ... You, Y.N. (2014). The increasing incidence of young-onset colorectal cancer: A call to action. *Mayo Clinic Proceedings, 89,* 216–224. https://doi.org/10.1016/j.mayocp.2013.09.006

Allegra, C.J., Rumble, R.B., & Schilsky, R.L. (2016). Extended *RAS* gene mutation testing in metastatic colorectal carcinoma to predict response to anti–epidermal growth factor receptor monoclonal antibody therapy: American Society of Clinical Oncology provisional clinical opinion update 2015 summary. *Journal of Oncology Practice, 12,* 180–181. https://doi.org/10.1200/JOP.2015.007898

André, T., Boni, C., Mounedji-Boudiaf, L., Navarro, M., Tabernero, J., Hickish, T., ... de Gramont, A. (2004). Oxaliplatin, fluorouracil, and leucovorin as adjuvant treatment for colon cancer. *New England Journal of Medicine, 350,* 2343–2351. https://doi.org/10.1056/NEJMoa032709

André, T., Boni, C., Navarro, M., Tabernero, J., Hickish, T., Topham, C., ... de Gramont, A. (2009). Improved overall survival with oxaliplatin, fluorouracil, and leucovorin as adjuvant treatment in stage II or III colon cancer in the MOSAIC trial. *Journal of Clinical Oncology, 27,* 3109–3116. https://doi.org/10.1200/JCO.2008.20.6771

Aune, D., Chan, D.S.M., Lau, R., Vieira, R., Greenwood, D.C., Kampman, E., & Norat, T. (2011). Dietary fibre, whole grains, and risk of colorectal cancer: Systematic review and dose-response meta-analysis of prospective studies. *BMJ, 343,* d6617. https://doi.org/10.1136/bmj.d6617

Bains, S.J., Mahic, M., Myklebust, T.Å., Småstuen, M.C., Yaqub, S., Dørum, L.M., ... Taskén, K. (2016). Aspirin as secondary prevention in patients with colorectal cancer: An unselected population-based study. *Journal of Clinical Oncology, 34,* 2501–2508. https://doi.org/10.1200/JCO.2015.65.3519

Bartelink, H., Roelofsen, F., Eschwege, F., Rougier, P., Bosset, J.F., Gonzalez, D.G., ... Pierart, M. (1997). Concomitant radiotherapy and chemotherapy is superior to radiotherapy alone in the treatment of locally advanced anal cancer: Results of a phase III randomized trial of the European Organization for Research and Treatment of Cancer Radiotherapy and Gastrointestinal Cooperative Groups. *Journal of Clinical Oncology, 15,* 2040–2049. https://doi.org/10.1200/JCO.1997.15.5.2040

Bendell, J.C., Kim, T.W., Goh, B.C., Wallin, J., Oh, D.-Y., Han, S.-W., ... Bang, Y.-J. (2016). Clinical activity and safety of cobimetinib (cobi) and atezolizumab in colorectal cancer (CRC). *Journal of Clinical Oncology, 34*(Suppl.), Abstract 3502. Retrieved from http://meetinglibrary.asco.org/record/123622/abstract

Bentzen, A.G., Balteskard, L., Wanderås, E.H., Frykholm, G., Wilsgaard, T., Dahl, O., & Guren, M.G. (2013). Impaired health-related quality of life after chemoradiotherapy for anal cancer: Late effects in a national cohort of 128 survivors. *Acta Oncologica, 52,* 736–744. https://doi.org/10.3109/0284186X.2013.770599

Biagi, J.J., Raphael, M.J., Mackillop, W.J., Kong, W., King, W.D., & Booth, C.M. (2011). Association between time to initiation of adjuvant chemotherapy and survival in colorectal cancer: A systematic review and meta-analysis. *JAMA, 305,* 2335–2342. https://doi.org/10.1001/jama.2011.749

Bibbins-Domingo, K. (2016). Aspirin use for the primary prevention of cardiovascular disease and colorectal cancer: U.S. Preventive Services Task Force recommendation statement. *Annals of Internal Medicine, 164,* 836–845. https://doi.org/10.7326/M16-0577

Bonadona, V., Bonaïti, B., Olschwang, S., Grandjouan, S., Huiart, L., Longy, M., ... Bonaïti-Pellié, C. (2011). Cancer risks associated with germline mutations in *MLH1, MSH2,* and *MSH6* genes in Lynch syndrome. *JAMA, 305,* 2304–2310. https://doi.org/10.1001/jama.2011.743

Boyle, T., Keegel, T., Bull, F., Heyworth, J., & Fritschi, L. (2012). Physical activity and risks of proximal and distal colon cancers: A systematic review and meta-analysis. *Journal of the National Cancer Institute, 104,* 1548–1561. https://doi.org/10.1093/jnci/djs354

Brenner, H., Chang-Claude, J., Seiler, C.M., Stürmer, T., & Hoffmeister, M. (2007). Potential for colorectal cancer prevention of sigmoidoscopy versus colonoscopy: Population-based case control study. *Cancer Epidemiology, Biomarkers and Prevention, 16,* 494–499. https://doi.org/10.1158/1055-9965.EPI-06-0460

Burn, J., Gerdes, A.-M, Macrae, F., Mecklin, J.-P., Moeslein, G., Olschwang, S., ... Bishop, D.T. (2011). Long-term effect of aspirin on cancer risk in carriers of hereditary colorectal cancer: An analysis from the CAPP2 randomised controlled trial. *Lancet, 378,* 2081–2087. https://doi.org/10.1016/S0140-6736(11)61049-0

Burt, R., & Neklason, D.W. (2005). Genetic testing for inherited colon cancer. *Gastroenterology, 128,* 1696–1716. https://doi.org/10.1053/j.gastro.2005.03.036

Campbell, P.T., Patel, A.V., Newton, C.C., Jacobs, E.J., & Gapstur, S.M. (2013). Associations of recreational physical activity and leisure time spent sitting with colorectal cancer survival. *Journal of Clinical Oncology, 31,* 876–885. https://doi.org/10.1200/JCO.2012.45.9735

Cassidy, J., Clarke, S., Díaz-Rubio, E., Scheithauer, W., Figer, A., Wong, R., ... Saltz, L. (2008). Randomized phase III study of capecitabine plus oxaliplatin compared with fluorouracil/folinic acid plus oxaliplatin as first-line therapy for metastatic colorectal cancer. *Journal of Clinical Oncology, 26,* 2006–2012. https://doi.org/10.1200/JCO.2007.14.9898

Chan, A.T., & Giovannucci, E.L. (2010). Primary prevention of colorectal cancer. *Gastroenterology, 138,* 2029–2043.e10. https://doi.org/10.1053/j.gastro.2010.01.057

Chiao, E.Y., Giordano, T.P., Palefsky, J.M., Tyring, S., & Serag, H.E. (2006). HIV/AIDS: Screening HIV-infected individuals for anal cancer precursor lesions: A systematic review. *Clinical Infectious Diseases, 43,* 223–233. https://doi.org/10.1086/505219

Chung, M., Lee, J., Terasawa, T., Lau, J., & Trikalinos, T.A. (2011). Vitamin D with or without calcium supplementation for prevention of cancer and fractures: An updated meta-analysis for the U.S. Preventive Services Task Force. *Annals of Internal Medicine, 155,* 827–838. https://doi.org/10.7326/0003-4819-155-12-201112200-00005

Compton, C.C., Fielding, L.P., Burgart, L.J., Conley, B., Cooper, H.S., Hamilton, S.R., … Willett, C. (2000). Prognostic factors in colorectal cancer. *Archives of Pathology and Laboratory Medicine, 124,* 979–994.

Czito, B.G., Ahmed, S., Kalady, M., & Eng, C. (2015). Cancer of the anal region. In V.T. DeVita Jr., T.S. Lawrence, & S.A. Rosenberg (Eds.), *DeVita, Hellman, and Rosenberg's cancer: Principles and practice of oncology* (10th ed., pp. 842–856). Philadelphia, PA: Wolters Kluwer Health.

Daling, J.R., Madeleine, M.M., Johnson, L.G., Schwartz, S.M., Shera, K.A., Wurscher, M.A., … McDougall, J.K. (2004). Human papillomavirus, smoking, and sexual practices in the etiology of anal cancer. *Cancer, 101,* 270–280. https://doi.org/10.1002/cncr.20365

Deng, G., Bell, I., Crawley, S., Gum, J., Terdiman, J.P., Allen, B.A., … Kim, Y.S. (2004). *BRAF* mutation is frequently present in sporadic colorectal cancer with methylated hMLH1, but not in hereditary nonpolyposis colorectal cancer. *Clinical Cancer Research, 10,* 191–195. https://doi.org/10.1158/1078-0432.CCR-1118-3

Deutsch, E., Lemanski, C., Pignon, J.P., Levy, A., Delarochefordiere, A., Martel-Lafay, I., … Azria, D. (2013). Unexpected toxicity of cetuximab combined with conventional chemoradiotherapy in patients with locally advanced anal cancer: Results of the Unicancer Accord 16 phase II trial. *Annals of Oncology, 24,* 2834–2838. https://doi.org/10.1093/annonc/mdt368

Ekbom, A., Helmick, C., Zack, M., & Adami, H.-O. (1990). Ulcerative colitis and colorectal cancer—A population-based study. *New England Journal of Medicine, 323,* 1228–1233. https://doi.org/10.1056/NEJM199011013231802

Eng, C., Chang, G.J., You, Y.N., Das, P., Rodriguez-Bigas, M., Xing, Y., … Wolff, R.A. (2014). The role of systemic chemotherapy and multidisciplinary management in improving the overall survival of patients with metastatic squamous cell carcinoma of the anal canal. *Oncotarget, 5,* 11133–11142. https://doi.org/10.18632/oncotarget.2563

Feight, D., Baney, T., Bruce, S., & McQuestion, M. (2011). Putting evidence into practice: Evidence-based interventions for radiation dermatitis. *Clinical Journal of Oncology Nursing, 15,* 481–492. https://doi.org/10.1188/11.CJON.481-492

Flam, M., John, M., Pajak, T.F., Petrelli, N., Myerson, R., Doggett, S., … Murray, K. (1996). Role of mitomycin in combination with fluorouracil and radiotherapy, and of salvage chemoradiation in the definitive nonsurgical treatment of epidermoid carcinoma of the anal canal: Results of a phase III randomized intergroup study. *Journal of Clinical Oncology, 14,* 2527–2539. https://doi.org/10.1200/jco.1996.14.9.2527

Fokas, E., Liersch, T., Fietkau, R., Hohenberger, W., Beissbarth, T., Hess, C., … Rödel, C. (2014). Tumor regression grading after preoperative chemoradiotherapy for locally advanced rectal carcinoma revisited: Updated results of the CAO/ARO/AIO-94 trial. *Journal of Clinical Oncology, 32,* 1554–1562. https://doi.org/10.1200/JCO.2013.54.3769

French, A.J., Sargent, D.J., Burgart, L.J., Foster, N.R., Kabat, B.F., Goldberg, R., … Thibodeau, S.N. (2008). Prognostic significance of defective mismatch repair and BRAF V600E in patients with colon cancer. *Clinical Cancer Research, 14,* 3408–3415. https://doi.org/10.1158/1078-0432.CCR-07-1489

Frisch, M. (2000). Human papillomavirus–associated cancers in patients with human immunodeficiency virus infection and acquired immunodeficiency syndrome. *Journal of the National Cancer Institute, 92,* 1500–1510. https://doi.org/10.1093/jnci/92.18.1500

Genentech, Inc. (2018). *Avastin® (bevacizumab)* [Package insert]. Retrieved from https://www.gene.com/download/pdf/avastin_prescribing.pdf

Giuliano, A.R., Palefsky, J.M., Goldstone, S., Moreira, E.D., Penny, M.E., Aranda, C., … Guris, D. (2011). Efficacy of quadrivalent HPV vaccine against HPV infection and disease in males. *New England Journal of Medicine, 364,* 401–411. https://doi.org/10.1056/NEJMoa0909537

Glynne-Jones, R., Meadows, H., Wan, S., Gollins, S., Leslie, M., Levine, E., ... Sebag-Montefiore, D. (2008). EXTRA—A multicenter phase II study of chemoradiation using a 5 day per week oral regimen of capecitabine and intravenous mitomycin C in anal cancer. *International Journal of Radiation Oncology, Biology, Physics, 72,* 119–126. https://doi.org/10.1016/j.ijrobp.2007.12.012

Grothey, A., Van Cutsem, E., Sobrero, A., Siena, S., Falcone, A., Ychou, M., ... Laurent, D. (2013). Regorafenib monotherapy for previously treated metastatic colorectal cancer (CORRECT): An international, multicentre, randomised, placebo-controlled, phase 3 trial. *Lancet, 381,* 303–312. https://doi.org/10.1016/S0140-6736(12)61900-X

Gunderson, L.L., Moughan, J., Ajani, J.A., Pedersen, J.E., Winter, K.A., Benson, A.B., III, ... Willett, C.G. (2013). Anal carcinoma: Impact of TN category of disease on survival, disease relapse, and colostomy failure in US Gastrointestinal Intergroup RTOG 98-11 phase 3 trial. *International Journal of Radiation Oncology, Biology, Physics, 87,* 638–645. https://doi.org/10.1016/j.ijrobp.2013.07.035

Hamilton, W., Round, A., Sharp, D., & Peters, T.J. (2005). Clinical features of colorectal cancer before diagnosis: A population-based case–control study. *British Journal of Cancer, 93,* 399–405. https://doi.org/10.1038/sj.bjc.6602714

Hendriks, Y.M.C., de Jong, A.E., Morreau, H., Tops, C.M.J., Vasen, H.F., Wijnen, J.T., ... Bröcker-Vriends, A.H.J.T. (2006). Diagnostic approach and management of Lynch syndrome (hereditary nonpolyposis colorectal carcinoma): A guide for clinicians. *CA: A Cancer Journal for Clinicians, 56,* 213–225. https://doi.org/10.3322/canjclin.56.4.213

Henley, S.J., Singh, S.D., King, J., Wilson, R.J., O'Neil, M.E., & Ryerson, A.B. (2015). Invasive cancer incidence and survival—United States, 2012. *Morbidity and Mortality Weekly Report, 64,* 1353–1358. https://doi.org/10.15585/mmwr.mm6449a1

Hershman, D.L., Lacchetti, C., & Loprinzi, C.L. (2014). Prevention and management of chemotherapy-induced peripheral neuropathy in survivors of adult cancers: American Society of Clinical Oncology clinical practice guideline summary. *Journal of Oncology Practice, 10,* e421–e424. https://doi.org/10.1200/JOP.2014.001776

Hewitt, M., Greenfield, S., & Stovall, E. (Eds.). (2006). *From cancer patient to cancer survivor: Lost in transition.* Retrieved from https://www.nap.edu/catalog/11468/from-cancer-patient-to-cancer-survivor-lost-in-transition

Hofheinz, R., Gencer, D., Schulz, H., Stahl, M., Hegewisch-Becker, S., Loeffler, L.M., ... Schneeweiss, A. (2015). Mapisal versus urea cream as prophylaxis for capecitabine-associated hand-foot syndrome: A randomized phase III trial of the AIO Quality of Life Working Group. *Journal of Clinical Oncology, 33,* 2444–2449. https://doi.org/10.1200/JCO.2014.60.4587

Jackson, L.K., Johnson, D.B., Sosman, J.A., Murphy, B.A., & Epstein, J.B. (2015). Oral health in oncology: Impact of immunotherapy. *Supportive Care in Cancer, 23,* 1–3. https://doi.org/10.1007/s00520-014-2434-6

James, R.D., Glynne-Jones, R., Meadows, H.M., Cunningham, D., Myint, A.S., Saunders, M.P., ... Sebag-Montefiore, D. (2013). Mitomycin or cisplatin chemoradiation with or without maintenance chemotherapy for treatment of squamous-cell carcinoma of the anus (ACT II): A randomised, phase 3, open-label, 2×2 factorial trial. *Lancet Oncology, 14,* 516–524. https://doi.org/10.1016/S1470-2045(13)70086-X

Jemal, A., Bray, F., Center, M.M., Ferlay, J., Ward, E., & Forman, D. (2011). Global cancer statistics. *CA: A Cancer Journal for Clinicians, 61,* 69–90. https://doi.org/10.3322/caac.20107

Jessup, J.M., Goldberg, R.M., Asare, E.A., Benson, A.B., III, Brierley, J.D., Chang, G.J., ... Washington, M.K. (2017). Colon and rectum. In M.B. Amin (Ed.), *AJCC cancer staging manual* (8th ed., pp. 251–274). Chicago, IL: Springer.

Jones, M., Hruby, G., Solomon, M., Rutherford, N., & Martin, J. (2015). The role of FDG-PET in the initial staging and response assessment of anal cancer: A systematic review and meta-analysis. *Annals of Surgical Oncology, 22,* 3574–3581. https://doi.org/10.1245/s10434-015-4391-9

Kanas, G.P., Taylor, A., Primrose, J.N., Langeberg, W.J., Kelsh, M.A., Mowat, F.S., ... Poston, G. (2012). Survival after liver resection in metastatic colorectal cancer: Review and meta-analysis of prognostic factors. *Clinical Epidemiology, 283,* 283–301. https://doi.org/10.2147/CLEP.S34285

Kanemitsu, Y., Kato, T., Hirai, T., Yasui, K., Morimoto, T., Shimizu, Y., ... Yamamura, Y. (2003). Survival after curative resection for mucinous adenocarcinoma of the colorectum. *Diseases of the Colon and Rectum, 46,* 160–167. https://doi.org/10.1007/s10350-004-6518-0

Karahalios, A., English, D.R., & Simpson, J.A. (2015). Weight change and risk of colorectal cancer: A systematic review and meta-analysis. *American Journal of Epidemiology, 181,* 832–845. https://doi.org/10.1093/aje/kwu357

Kenig, J., & Richter, P. (2013). Definition of the rectum and level of the peritoneal reflection—Still a matter of debate? *Videosurgery and Other Miniinvasive Techniques, 3,* 183–186. https://doi.org/10.5114/wiitm.2011.34205

Knijn, N., Mogk, S.C., Teerenstra, S., Simmer, F., & Nagtegaal, I.D. (2016). Perineural invasion is a strong prognostic factor in colorectal cancer: A systematic review. *American Journal of Surgical Pathology, 40,* 103–112. https://doi.org/10.1097/PAS.0000000000000518

Koopman, M., Kortman, G.A.M., Mekenkamp, L., Ligtenberg, M.J.L., Hoogerbrugge, N., Antonini, N.F., ... van Krieken, J.H.J.M. (2009). Deficient mismatch repair system in patients with sporadic advanced colorectal cancer. *British Journal of Cancer, 100,* 266–273. https://doi.org/10.1038/sj.bjc.6604867

Lacouture, M.E., Mitchell, E.P., Piperdi, B., Pillai, M.V., Shearer, H., Iannotti, N., ... Yassine, M. (2010). Skin toxicity evaluation protocol with panitumumab (STEPP), a phase II, open-label, randomized trial evaluating the impact of a pre-emptive skin treatment regimen on skin toxicities and quality of life in patients with metastatic colorectal cancer. *Journal of Clinical Oncology, 28,* 1351–1357. https://doi.org/10.1200/JCO.2008.21.7828

Lanza, G., Gafà, R., Santini, A., Maestri, I., Guerzoni, L., & Cavazzini, L. (2006). Immunohistochemical test for MLH1 and MSH2 expression predicts clinical outcome in stage II and III colorectal cancer patients. *Journal of Clinical Oncology, 24,* 2359–2367. https://doi.org/10.1200/JCO.2005.03.2433

Le, D.T., Uram, J.N., Wang, H., Bartlett, B.R., Kemberling, H., Eyring, A.D., ... Diaz, L.A., Jr. (2015). PD-1 blockade in tumors with mismatch-repair deficiency. *New England Journal of Medicine, 372,* 2509–2520. https://doi.org/10.1056/NEJMoa1500596

Le, D.T., Uram, J.N., Wang, H., Bartlett, B.R., Kemberling, A., Eyring, A.D., ... Diaz, L.A. (2016). Programmed death-1 blockade in mismatch repair deficient colorectal cancer. *Journal of Clinical Oncology, 34*(Suppl. 15), 103. Retrieved from http://ascopubs.org/doi/abs/10.1200/JCO.2016.34.15_suppl.103

Lester, J. (2018). Surgical oncology. In C.H. Yarbro, D. Wujcik, & B.H. Gobel (Eds.), *Cancer nursing: Principles and practice* (8th ed., pp. 243–262). Burlington, MA: Jones & Bartlett Learning.

Levin, B., Lieberman, D.A., McFarland, B., Smith, R.A., Brooks, D., Andrews, K.S., ... Winawer, S.J. (2008). Screening and surveillance for the early detection of colorectal cancer and adenomatous polyps, 2008: A joint guideline from the American Cancer Society, the US Multi-Society Task Force on Colorectal Cancer, and the American College of Radiology. *CA: A Cancer Journal for Clinicians, 58,* 130–160. https://doi.org/10.3322/CA.2007.0018

Libutti, S.K., Saltz, L.B., Willett, C.G., & Levine, R.A. (2015). Cancer of the colon. In V.T. DeVita Jr., T.S. Lawrence, & S.A. Rosenberg (Eds.), *DeVita, Hellman, and Rosenberg's cancer: Principles and practice of oncology* (10th ed., pp. 768–812). Philadelphia, PA: Wolters Kluwer Health.

Lim, S.-B., Yu, C.S., Jang, S.J., Kim, T.W., Kim, J.H., & Kim, J.C. (2010). Prognostic significance of lymphovascular invasion in sporadic colorectal cancer. *Diseases of the Colon and Rectum, 53,* 377–384. https://doi.org/10.1007/DCR.0b013e3181cf8ae5

Lynch, H.T., & Chapelle, A.D. (2003). Hereditary colorectal cancer. *New England Journal of Medicine, 348,* 919–932. https://doi.org/10.1056/NEJMra012242

Martinez, M.E., Jacobs, E.T., Ashbeck, E.L., Sinha, R., Lance, P., Alberts, D.S., & Thompson, P.A. (2007). Meat intake, preparation methods, mutagens and colorectal adenoma recurrence. *Carcinogenesis, 28,* 2019–2027. https://doi.org/10.1093/carcin/bgm179

Mayer, R.J., Van Cutsem, E., Falcone, A., Yoshino, T., Garcia-Carbonero, R., Mizunuma, N., ... Ohtsu, A. (2015). Randomized trial of TAS-102 for refractory metastatic colorectal cancer. *New England Journal of Medicine, 372,* 1909–1919. https://doi.org/10.1056/NEJMoa1414325

Meyerhardt, J.A., Mangu, P.B., Flynn, P.J., Korde, L., Loprinzi, C.L., Minsky, B.D., ... Benson, A.B., III. (2013). Follow-up care, surveillance protocol, and secondary prevention measures for survivors of colorectal cancer: American Society of Clinical Oncology clinical practice guideline endorsement. *Journal of Clinical Oncology, 31,* 4465–4470. https://doi.org/10.1200/JCO.2013.50.7442

Meyerhardt, J.A., Niedzwiecki, D., Hollis, D., Saltz, L.B., Hu, F.B., Mayer, R.J., ... Fuchs, C.S. (2007). Association of dietary patterns with cancer recurrence and survival in patients with stage III colon cancer. *JAMA, 298,* 754–764. https://doi.org/10.1001/jama.298.7.754

Moreno, C.C., Mittal, P.K., Sullivan, P.S., Rutherford, R., Staley, C.A., Cardona, K., ... Votaw, J.R. (2016). Colorectal cancer initial diagnosis: Screening colonoscopy, diagnostic colonoscopy, or emergent surgery, and tumor stage and size at initial presentation. *Clinical Colorectal Cancer, 15,* 67–73. https://doi.org/10.1016/j.clcc.2015.07.004

Mork, M., Hubosky, S.G., Rouprêt, M., Margulis, V., Raman, J., Lotan, Y., ... Matin, S.F. (2015). Lynch syndrome: A primer for urologists and panel recommendations. *Journal of Urology, 194,* 21–29. https://doi.org/10.1016/j.juro.2015.02.081

Morris, L., Do, V., Chard, J., & Brand, A.H. (2017). Radiation-induced vaginal stenosis: Current perspectives. *International Journal of Women's Health, 9,* 273–279. https://doi.org/10.2147/IJWH.S106796

Morris, V.K., Salem, M.E., Nimeiri, H., Iqbal, S., Singh, P., Ciombor, K., ... Eng, C. (2017). Nivolumab for previously treated unresectable metastatic anal cancer (NCI9673): A multicentre, single-arm, phase 2 study. *Lancet Oncology, 18,* 446–453. https://doi.org/10.1016/S1470-2045(17)30104-3

Moscicki, A., Hills, N.K., Shiboski, S., Darragh, T.M., Jay, N., & Palefsky, J. (1999). Risk factors for abnormal anal cytology in young heterosexual women. *Cancer Epidemiology, Biomarkers and Prevention, 8,* 173–178.

Mulder, S.A., Kranse, R., Damhuis, R.A., Wilt, J.H., Ouwendijk, R.J., Kuipers, E.J., & Leerdam, M.E. (2011). Prevalence and prognosis of synchronous colorectal cancer: A Dutch population-based study. *Cancer Epidemiology, 35,* 442–447. https://doi.org/10.1016/j.canep.2010.12.007

Nagore, E., Insa, A., & Sanmartin, O. (2000). Antineoplastic therapy–induced palmar plantar erythrodysesthesia ("hand-foot") syndrome: Incidence, recognition and management. *American Journal of Clinical Dermatology, 1,* 225–234. https://doi.org/10.2165/00128071-200001040-00004

Naidoo, J., Page, D.B., Li, B.T., Connell, L.C., Schindler, K., Lacouture, M.E., ... Wolchok, J.D. (2015). Toxicities of the anti-PD-1 and anti-PD-L1 immune checkpoint antibodies. *Annals of Oncology, 383,* 2375–2391. https://doi.org/10.1093/annonc/mdv383

National Comprehensive Cancer Network. (2018a). *NCCN Clinical Practice Guidelines in Oncology (NCCN Guidelines®): Anal carcinoma* [v.2.2018]. Retrieved from https://www.nccn.org/professionals/physician_gls/pdf/anal.pdf

National Comprehensive Cancer Network. (2018b). *NCCN Clinical Practice Guidelines in Oncology (NCCN Guidelines®): Colon cancer* [v.2.2018]. Retrieved from https://www.nccn.org/professionals/physician_gls/pdf/colon.pdf

National Comprehensive Cancer Network. (2018c). *NCCN Clinical Practice Guidelines in Oncology (NCCN Guidelines®): Genetic/familial high-risk assessment: Colorectal* [v.1.2018]. Retrieved from https://www.nccn.org/professionals/physician_gls/pdf/genetics_colon.pdf

National Comprehensive Cancer Network. (2018d). *NCCN Clinical Practice Guidelines in Oncology (NCCN Guidelines®): Rectal cancer* [v.1.2018]. Retrieved from https://www.nccn.org/professionals/physician_gls/pdf/rectal.pdf

Nelson, R.A., Levine, A.M., Bernstein, L., Smith, D.D., & Lai, L.L. (2013). Changing patterns of anal canal carcinoma in the United States. *Journal of Clinical Oncology, 31,* 1569–1575. https://doi.org/10.1200/JCO.2012.45.2524

Nicholson, B.D., Shinkins, B., Pathiraja, I., Roberts, N.W., James, T.J., Mallett, S., ... Mant, D. (2015). Blood CEA levels for detecting recurrent colorectal cancer. *Cochrane Database of Systematic Reviews, 2015*(12). https://doi.org/10.1002/14651858.CD011134.pub2

Orlich, M.J., Singh, P.N., Sabaté, J., Fan, J., Sveen, L., Bennett, H., ... Fraser, G.E. (2015). Vegetarian dietary patterns and the risk of colorectal cancers. *JAMA Internal Medicine, 175,* 767–776. http://doi.org/10.1001/jamainternmed.2015.59

Overman, M.J., McDermott, R., Leach, J.L., Lonardi, S., Lenz, H.-J., Morse, M.A., ... André, T. (2017). Nivolumab in patients with metastatic DNA mismatch repair-deficient or microsatellite instability-high colorectal cancer (CheckMate 142): An open-label, multicentre, phase 2 study. *Lancet Oncology, 18,* 1182–1191. https://doi.org/10.1016/S1470-2045(17)30422-9

Pachman, D.R., Qin, R., Seisler, D.K., Smith, E.M.L., Beutler, A.S., Ta, L.E., ... Loprinzi, C.L. (2015). Clinical course of oxaliplatin-induced neuropathy: Results from the randomized phase III trial N08CB (Alliance). *Journal of Clinical Oncology, 33,* 3416–3422. http://doi.org/10.1200/JCO.2014.58.8533

Palefsky, J.M., Giuliano, A.R., Goldstone, S., Moreira, E.D., Aranda, C., Jessen, H., ... Garner, E.I. (2011). HPV vaccine against anal HPV infection and anal intraepithelial neoplasia. *New England Journal of Medicine, 365,* 1576–1585. https://doi.org/10.1056/NEJMoa1010971

Palomaki, G.E., McClain, M.R., Melillo, S., Hampel, H.L., & Thibodeau, S.N. (2009). EGAPP supplementary evidence review: DNA testing strategies aimed at reducing morbidity and mortality from Lynch syndrome. *Genetics in Medicine, 11,* 42–65. https://doi.org/10.1097/GIM.0b013e31818fa2db

Pfizer Inc. (2016). *Camptosar® (irinotecan)* [Package insert]. Retrieved from http://labeling.pfizer.com/ShowLabeling.aspx?id=533

Pietrantonio, F., Garassino, M.C., Torri, V., & Braud, F.D. (2012). Reply to FOLFIRI plus cetuximab versus FOLFIRI plus bevacizumab as first-line treatment for patients with metastatic colorectal cancer-subgroup analysis of patients with KRAS-mutated tumours in the randomised German AIO study KRK-0306. *Annals of Oncology, 23,* 2771–2772. https://doi.org/10.1093/annonc/mds332

Pino, M.S., & Chung, D.C. (2010). The chromosomal instability pathway in colon cancer. *Gastroenterology, 138,* 2059–2072. https://doi.org/10.1053/j.gastro.2009.12.065

Plummer, J.M., Leake, P.-A., & Albert, M.R. (2017). Recent advances in the management of rectal cancer: No surgery, minimal surgery or minimally invasive surgery. *World Journal of Gastrointestinal Surgery, 9,* 139–148. https://doi.org/10.4240/wjgs.v9.i6.139

Popat, S., Hubner, R., & Houlston, R.S. (2005). Systematic review of microsatellite instability and colorectal cancer prognosis. *Journal of Clinical Oncology, 23,* 609–618. https://doi.org/10.1001/jama.2013.285718

Primrose, J.N., Perera, R., Gray, A., Rose, P., Fuller, A., Corkhill, A., ... Mant, D. (2014). Effect of 3 to 5 years of scheduled CEA and CT follow-up to detect recurrence of colorectal cancer. *JAMA, 311,* 263–270. https://doi.org/10.1001/jama.2013.285718

Ramsey, S.D., Berry, K., Moinpour, C., Giedzinska, A., & Andersen, M.R. (2002). Quality of life in long term survivors of colorectal cancer. *American Journal of Gastroenterology, 97,* 1228–1234. https://doi.org/10.1111/j.1572-0241.2002.05694.x

Rothwell, P.M., Wilson, M., Elwin, C., Norrving, B., Algra, A., Warlow, C.P., & Meade, T.W. (2010). Long-term effect of aspirin on colorectal cancer incidence and mortality: 20-year follow-up of five randomised trials. *Lancet, 376,* 1741–1750. https://doi.org/10.1016/S0140-6736(10)61543-7

Ruers, T., Van Coevorden, F., Punt, C.J.A., Pierie, J.-P.E.N., Borel-Rinkes, I., Ledermann, J.A., ... Nordlinger, B. (2017). Local treatment of unresectable colorectal liver metastases: Results of a randomized phase II trial. *Journal of the National Cancer Institute, 109,* djx015. https://doi.org/10.1093/jnci/djx015

Rutter, M.D. (2011). Surveillance programmes for neoplasia in colitis. *Journal of Gastroenterology, 46*(Suppl. 1), 1–5. https://doi.org/10.1007/s00535-010-0309-2

Ryan, D.P., Compton, C.C., & Mayer, R.J. (2000). Carcinoma of the anal canal. *New England Journal of Medicine, 342,* 792–800. https://doi.org/10.1056/NEJM200003163421107

Sagiv, E., Memeo, L., Karin, A., Kazanov, D., Jacob-Hirsch, J., Mansukhani, M., ... Arber, N. (2006). CD24 is a new oncogene, early at the multistep process of colorectal cancer carcinogenesis. *Gastroenterology, 131,* 630–639. https://doi.org/10.1053/j.gastro.2006.04.028

Sargent, D.J., Wieand, H.S., Haller, D.G., Gray, R., Benedetti, J.K., Buyse, M., ... De Gramont, A. (2005). Disease-free survival versus overall survival as a primary end point for adjuvant colon cancer studies: Individual patient data from 20,898 patients on 18 randomized trials. *Journal of Clinical Oncology, 23,* 8664–8670. https://doi.org/10.1200/JCO.2005.01.6071

Sauer, R., Becker, H., Hohenberger, W., Rödel, C., Wittekind, C., Fietkau, R., ... Raab, R. (2004). Preoperative versus postoperative chemoradiotherapy for rectal cancer. *New England Journal of Medicine, 351,* 1731–1740. https://doi.org/10.1056/NEJMoa040694

Schmeler, K.M., Lynch, H.T., Chen, L., Munsell, M.F., Soliman, P.T., Clark, M.B., ... Lu, K.H. (2006). Prophylactic surgery to reduce the risk of gynecologic cancers in the lynch syndrome. *New England Journal of Medicine, 354,* 261–269. https://doi.org/10.1056/NEJMoa052627

Schmid, D., & Leitzmann, M.F. (2014). Association between physical activity and mortality among breast cancer and colorectal cancer survivors: A systematic review and meta-analysis. *Annals of Oncology, 25,* 1293–1311. https://doi.org/10.1093/annonc/mdu012

Serup-Hansen, E., Linnemann, D., Skovrider-Ruminski, W., Høgdall, E., Geertsen, P.F., & Havsteen, H. (2014). Human papillomavirus genotyping and p16 expression as prognostic factors for patients with American Joint Committee on Cancer stages I to III carcinoma of the anal canal. *Journal of Clinical Oncology, 32,* 1812–1817. https://doi.org/10.1200/JCO.2013.52.3464

Shah, S.A., Haddad, R., Al-Sukhni, W., Kim, R.D., Grant, P.D., Taylor, B.R., & Wei, A.C. (2006). Surgical resection of hepatic and pulmonary metastases from colorectal carcinoma. *Journal of the American College of Surgeons, 202,* 468–475. https://doi.org/10.1016/j.jamcollsurg.2005.11.008

Shi, Q., Sobrero, A.F., Shields, A.F., Yoshino, T., Paul, J., Taieb, J., ... Iveson, T. (2017). Prospective pooled analysis of six phase III trials investigating duration of adjuvant (adjuv) oxaliplatin-based therapy (3 vs 6 months) for patients (pts) with stage III colon cancer (CC): The IDEA (International Duration Evaluation of Adjuvant Chemotherapy) collaboration. *Journal of Clinical Oncology, 35*(Suppl.), Abstract LBA1. Retrieved from http://meetinglibrary.asco.org/record/147028/abstract

Siegel, R.L., Fedewa, S.A., Anderson, W.F., Miller, K.D., Ma, J., Rosenberg, P.S., & Jemal, A. (2017). Colorectal cancer incidence patterns in the United States, 1974–2013. *Journal of the National Cancer Institute, 109*, djw322. https://doi.org/10.1093/jnci/djw322

Siegel, R.L., Miller, K.D., & Jemal, A. (2018). Cancer statistics, 2018. *CA: A Cancer Journal for Clinicians, 68*, 7–30. https://doi.org/10.3322/caac.21442

Siegel, R.L., Ward, E.M., & Jemal, A. (2012). Trends in colorectal cancer incidence rates in the United States by tumor location and stage, 1992–2008. *Cancer Epidemiology, Biomarkers and Prevention, 21*, 411–416. https://doi.org/10.1158/1055-9965.EPI-11-1020

Stern, J., & Ippoliti, C. (2003). Management of acute cancer treatment-induced diarrhea. *Seminars in Oncology Nursing, 19*, 11–16. https://doi.org/10.1053/j.soncn.2003.09.009

Taylor, D.P., Burt, R.W., Williams, M.S., Haug, P.J., & Cannon-Albright, L.A. (2010). Population-based family history–specific risks for colorectal cancer: A constellation approach. *Gastroenterology, 138*, 877–885. https://doi.org/10.1053/j.gastro.2009.11.044

Torre, L.A., Bray, F., Siegel, R.L., Ferlay, J., Lortet-Tieulent, J., & Jemal, A. (2015). Global cancer statistics, 2012. *CA: A Cancer Journal for Clinicians, 65*, 87–108. https://doi.org/10.3322/caac.21262

Van Cutsem, E., Köhne, C., Hitre, E., Zaluski, J., Chien, C.C., Makhson, A., ... Rougier, P. (2009). Cetuximab and chemotherapy as initial treatment for metastatic colorectal cancer. *New England Journal of Medicine, 360*, 1408–1417. https://doi.org/10.1056/NEJMoa0805019

Vasen, H.F., Watson, P., Mecklin, J.P., & Lynch, H.T. (1999). New clinical criteria for hereditary nonpolyposis colorectal cancer (HNPCC, Lynch syndrome) proposed by the International Collaborative Group on HNPCC. *Gastroenterology, 116*, 1453–1456.

Vinay, D.S., Ryan, E.P., Pawelec, G., Talib, W.H., Stagg, J., Elkord, E., ... Kwon, B.S. (2015). Immune evasion in cancer: Mechanistic basis and therapeutic strategies. *Seminars in Cancer Biology, 35*(Suppl.), S185–S198. https://doi.org/10.1016/j.semcancer.2015.03.004

Vogel, W.H. (2017). Sexuality alterations. In S. Newton, M. Hickey, & J.M. Brant (Eds.), *Mosby's oncology nursing advisor: A comprehensive guide to clinical practice* (2nd ed., pp. 347–349). St. Louis, MO: Elsevier.

Welton, M.L., Steele, S.R., Goodman, K.A., Gunderson, L.L., Asare, E.A., Brierley, J.D., ... Jessup, J.M. (2017). Anus. In M.B. Amin (Ed.), *AJCC cancer staging manual* (8th ed., pp. 275–284). Chicago, IL: Springer.

West, N.P., Hohenberger, W., Weber, K., Perrakis, A., Finan, P.J., & Quirke, P. (2010). Complete mesocolic excision with central vascular ligation produces an oncologically superior specimen compared with standard surgery for carcinoma of the colon. *Journal of Clinical Oncology, 28*, 272–278. https://doi.org/10.1200/JCO.2009.24.1448

Wilkes, G.M. (2018). Colon, rectal, and anal cancers. In C.H. Yarbro, D. Wujcik, & B.H. Gobel (Eds.), *Cancer nursing: Principles and practice* (8th ed., pp. 243–262). Burlington, MA: Jones & Bartlett Learning.

Zacharias, A.J., Jayakrishnan, T.T., Rajeev, R., Rilling, W.S., Thomas, J.P., George, B., ... Turaga, K.K. (2015). Comparative effectiveness of hepatic artery based therapies for unresectable colorectal liver metastases: A meta-analysis. *PLOS ONE, 10*. https://doi.org/10.1371/journal.pone.0139940

Zheng, Z., Jemal, A., Lin, C.C., Hu, C.-Y., & Chang, G.J. (2015). Comparative effectiveness of laparoscopy vs open colectomy among nonmetastatic colon cancer patients: An analysis using the National Cancer Data Base. *Journal of the National Cancer Institute, 107*, dju491. https://doi.org/10.1093/jnci/dju491

Zimmerer, T., Böcker, U., Wenz, F., & Singer, M.V. (2008). Medical prevention and treatment of acute and chronic radiation induced enteritis—Is there any proven therapy? A short review. *Zeitschrift für Gastroenterologie, 46*, 441–448. https://doi.org/10.1055/s-2008-1027150

CHAPTER 2

Esophageal Cancer

Laura A. Pachella, RN, MSN, AGPCNP-BC, AOCNP®

Introduction

Cancer of the esophagus is an important worldwide health problem because of its poor prognosis and its relatively high incidence in some parts of the world. Advances in surgical techniques, chemotherapy, and radiation therapy have not substantially modified its prognosis over the past 25 years. The aim of this chapter is to provide an update of the epidemiology, clinical features, pathogenetic mechanisms, and new diagnostic and therapeutic approaches for esophageal cancer.

Anatomy of the Esophagus

The esophagus is a muscular tube that begins as the continuation of the pharynx in the neck and ends at the junction with the stomach. It transports food and fluid from the oral cavity to the stomach through the thoracic cavity and passes through the diaphragmatic hiatus into the abdomen (Oezcelik & DeMeester, 2011). On occasion, the passage of gastric contents occurs in a retrograde fashion called vomiting (Rice & Bronner, 2011).

The average length of the esophagus, measured from the incisor teeth to the gastroesophageal junction (GEJ), is 22 cm in men and 21 cm in women (Oezcelik & DeMeester, 2011). The esophagus is described by two different classifications and divided into three different regions for each system. The first classification system is anatomic and comprises the cervical region, which is from 15–20 cm; the thoracic region, which is 25–40 cm; and the abdominal region, which is 40–45 cm. Variation exists in this system, as the length of the esophagus in each patient is unique. The second classification system uses the description of the location of the region. The upper third is from 15–25 cm, the middle third is from 25–30 cm, and the lower is third is from 30–45 cm, which also

Table 2-1. Sites of Esophageal Cancer

Location by Anatomic Markings	Location by Division of the Esophagus	Measurement (cm)
Cervical	Upper	15–20
	Upper	20–25
Thoracic	Middle	25–30
	Lower	30–40
Abdominal	Lower, gastroesophageal junction cardia	40–45

Note. Based on information from Oezcelik & DeMeester, 2011; Rice & Bronner, 2011.

extends into the GEJ cardia. These descriptors can be seen in endoscopy and imaging reports. The GEJ is the location where the esophagus joins the stomach and is denoted by pathologic findings and anatomic markings. The GEJ is defined in a variety of modalities by endoscopic, surgical, histologic, and pathologic findings.

The lower esophageal sphincter is near the GEJ; however, it is not a readily identifiable structure and can only be identified on manometry (Rice & Bronner, 2011). The lower esophageal sphincter relaxes at the initiation of a swallow and allows for the food bolus to pass into the stomach. It acts as the main barrier against gastric contents refluxing into the esophagus (Oezcelik & DeMeester, 2011).

The esophageal wall is composed of four layers: the mucosa, submucosa, muscularis propria, and adventitia (see Figure 2-1). Each contributes a different function to the role of the esophagus. It is important to understand the wall of the esophagus when discussing the staging of esophageal cancer.

Mucosa

The esophageal epithelium turnover is approximately 21 days, as it is exposed to fluids and food on a constant basis. The basement membrane anchors the epithelium to the lamina propria and isolates the epithelium from the remainder of the esophageal wall. Destruction of the basement membrane by malignant cells originating in the epithelium is the first step of cancer invasion and thus defines an invasive carcinoma, distinguishing it from high-grade dysplasia, or carcinoma in situ (Rice & Bronner, 2011).

The lamina propria is a thin layer of loose connective tissue containing a complex of collagen and elastin fibers. The lamina propria contains a network of endothelial-lined channels, with both capillaries and lymphatics. This layer of the mucosa provides intramucosal carcinoma with access to the bloodstream or lymphatic spread. This is a large reason that esophageal cancer has the potential for early metastasis (Rice & Bronner, 2011).

The muscularis mucosae is the longitudinal layer of smooth muscle. It is the thickest muscularis mucosae of the entire gastrointestinal (GI) tract. It is important to understand this when assessing the depth of invasive carcinoma into the esophageal wall. The role of the muscularis mucosae in swallowing is not completely understood; however, it may dictate the amount of dilation that can occur when a food bolus enters the esophagus (Rice & Bronner, 2011).

Submucosa

The submucosa is the loose connective tissue containing blood vessels, lymphatics, and submucosal glands. These glands produce acid, mucin, bicarbonate, water, electrolytes, epidermal growth factor, and prostaglandins. These products protect the epithelium from exposure to fluids, acids, and food (Rice & Bronner, 2011).

Muscularis Propria

The muscularis propria is an inner layer of circular fibers and an outer longitudinal layer, which is responsible for peristalsis. Peristalsis

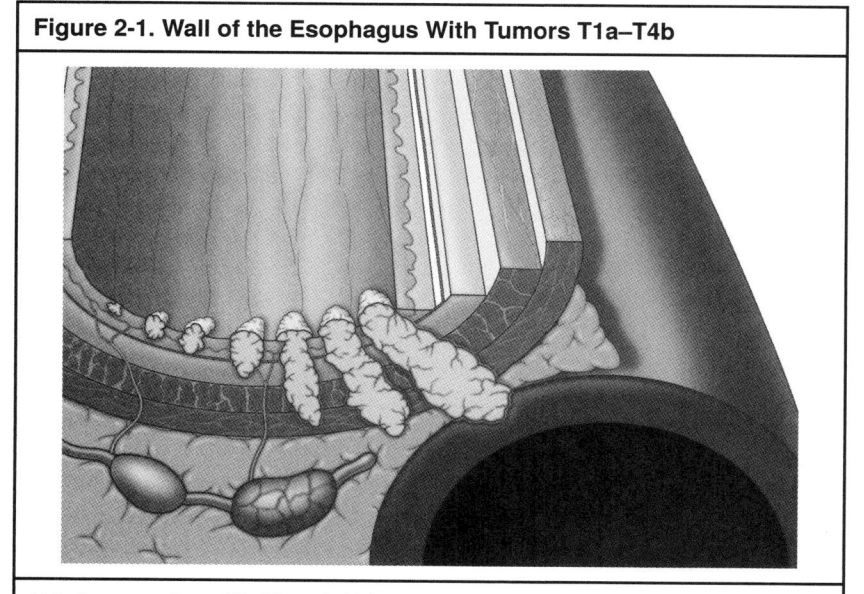

Figure 2-1. Wall of the Esophagus With Tumors T1a–T4b

Note. Image courtesy of Dr. Wayne L. Hofstetter. Used with permission.

is the involuntary wavelike contraction along the esophageal wall that forces along content inside the esophagus (Rice & Bronner, 2011).

Adventitia

The adventitia is the outermost layer of the esophageal wall. This fibrous layer covers the esophagus in a bed of fat, neurovascular and connective tissue, and elastin fibers (Oezcelik & DeMeester, 2011). The adventitia covers the esophagus and connects it to nearby structures. It also contains small vessels, lymphatic channels, and nerve fibers.

The anatomy of the esophagus is unique in that the lymphatics, vessels, and nerves are greatly interconnected with other associated organs because there is not a mesentery. This leads to the high rate of distant metastasis, as the esophagus is directly connected to these organs (Rice & Bronner, 2011).

Incidence and Epidemiology

Esophageal cancer is relatively rare in the United States. According to data from the American Cancer Society (2018), an estimated 17,290 new cases will be diagnosed in 2018, which represents 1% of all new cancers. An estimated 15,850 deaths from esophageal cancer will occur in the United States in 2018, which represents 2.6% of all cancer deaths. Patients are most commonly diagnosed between the ages of 65 and 74. In North America, esophageal cancer is seven times more common in men than women (Malhotra et al., 2017). Globally, esophageal cancer is the eighth most common cancer, with a higher incidence noted in Asia and Africa (Malhotra et al., 2017).

Etiology and Risk Factors

Esophageal cancer has two main histologic subtypes: adenocarcinoma and squamous cell carcinoma (SCC). The distinction is important when discussing the pathology and risk factors for the disease, as it dictates the treatment and workup.

Esophageal Adenocarcinoma

Esophageal adenocarcinoma (EAC) has been directly related to gastroesophageal reflux, specifically with weekly symptoms and obesity. EAC is more common than SCC in the Western hemisphere. Obesity rates have increased in the Western world, which has been correlated with an increase in rates of EAC. The exact link between obesity and EAC is not clear; however, an obese individual has a fivefold increased risk of developing EAC. This may be the result of increased intra-abdominal pressure secondary to central adiposity, which facilitates gastroesophageal reflux disease (GERD) and esophagitis, which predisposes for Barrett's esophagus (BE). Obesity as an independent risk factor is known to have carcinogenic effects via hormonal imbalance (Abbas & Krasna, 2017).

BE is a condition identified on endoscopy that appears as abnormal tongues of salmon-colored mucosa. The pathologic findings of BE identify intestinal metaplasia related to inflammation that can progress to low-grade dysplasia, high-grade dysplasia, and EAC. The rate of BE is 10%–15% in patients with a diagnosis of GERD. In the Western world, the prevalence of GERD is 10%–20% for the general population (Kethman & Hawn, 2017). Risk factors for BE include GERD, male sex, increasing age, central adiposity, family history of dysplastic BE or EAC, and smoking. Hiatal hernias and esophagitis have been associated with an increased risk of BE progressing to EAC. The 10-year cumulative risk of developing EAC is stratified to the degree of dysplasia. In the absence of dysplasia, the risk of EAC is 3%–6%; in the presence of low-grade dysplasia, 7%–13% of patients will develop EAC. High-grade dysplasia can be a concurrent diagnosis with microscopic adenocarcinoma in up to 40% of cases (Abbas & Krasna, 2017). BE is typically diagnosed on routine endoscopy for GERD or other esophageal or gastric issues. It is possible to develop BE without symptoms of GERD, as this is reported in 15%–45% of patients (Zakko, Lutzke, & Wang, 2017). Treatment for high-grade dysplasia in the esophagus includes serial endoscopy with radiofrequency ablation to eradicate premalignant cells.

Evidence supports that BE is an adaptation to the environment of high acid and bile and swallowed tobacco; many cases of benign BE metaplasia exist (Reid, 2017). It is important to highlight that many patients will not progress to EAC. The goal of detecting BE is to find patients who are at high risk for the development of EAC and to intervene early in the disease course or in the premalignancy phase. This would decrease the mortality from EAC and improve quality of life in the long run for patients (Reid, 2017).

Squamous Cell Carcinoma

SCC is the most common esophageal subtype in the world and is more commonly found outside of the Western hemisphere. Major risk factors include smoking tobacco and excessive alcohol intake. China has the highest consumption of cigarettes and also one of the highest incidences of SCC in the world (Malhotra et al., 2017). The chewing of betel quid and areca nut, which is a plant that can be mixed with tobacco, and the ingestion of teas with tannins are linked to a higher incidence of esophageal cancer (Zakko et al., 2017). Exposure to wood burning for heating of homes and cooking has been associated with higher incidence, as has high ingestion of foods containing nitrogenous products (Zakko et al., 2017).

A small but true risk of developing a secondary SCC in the esophagus also exists for patients who previously underwent radiation to the thorax for other malignancies. Patients who received radiation for Hodgkin lymphoma are at an increased risk for developing SCC, typically occurring at least 12 years after the radiation therapy (Morton et al., 2014). Patients with breast cancer who underwent mastectomy followed by adjuvant radiation were at a moderately increased risk of developing SCC beginning five years after radiation therapy and continuing throughout follow-up (Zablotska, Chak, Das, & Neugut, 2005). The patient's full history and any prior radiation treatments are an important part of history taking. In patients who have a history of radiation to the thorax, healthcare providers should have a low threshold to fully investigate any swallowing or other esophageal complaints with endoscopy (Morton et al., 2014).

Signs and Symptoms

Patients often present with a cluster of symptoms (see Figure 2-2), including dysphagia, which is defined as difficulty swallowing. Dysphagia requires close assessment to determine what types of foods specifically cause the patient to have difficulty swallowing. This is assessed by reporting dysphagia to solids, soft foods, or liquids. Patients may report progressive dysphagia and over time be able to eat less and less. Odynophagia, which is pain with swallowing, is often reported with dysphagia. Patients commonly present with weight loss. In some cases, the loss may just be a few pounds, whereas in others, the amount may be significant, and patients may present with signs of malnutrition and dehydration.

Figure 2-2. Signs and Symptoms of Esophageal Cancer

- Abdominal or chest pain
- Aspiration pneumonia
- Asymptomatic—early tumors
- Dysphagia
- Gastrointestinal bleed
- Odynophagia
- Regurgitation
- Weight loss

Regurgitation of food is reported when the tumor is too large to allow food to pass through the lumen of the esophagus. Aspiration pneumonia may develop if patients are frequently coughing and regurgitating food. Upper GI bleeding is also possible with regurgitation, particularly in gastric cardia tumors. Abdominal and chest pain will be present in patients with large tumors, which may press on adjacent organs, or in the setting of metastatic disease. Patients with early intraluminal tumors may be asymptomatic and without classic symptoms of the disease.

Diagnostic Evaluation

Diagnosis of esophageal cancer is most frequently made on endoscopy, possibly incidentally if the patient has a history of BE or other esophagitis and pathology reveals malignancy. The tumor can also be identified through patient-reported symptoms of dysphagia that prompt endoscopy, during which a malignancy is found. Imaging studies, including a computed tomography (CT) of the chest and abdomen with contrast, are necessary to assess the size of the tumor and to determine if metastatic disease or regional spread is present (Abbas & Krasna, 2017). If the tumor is small and early stage, it may not be seen on imaging at all. National Comprehensive Cancer Network® (NCCN®, 2018) guidelines recommend a positron-emission tomography–computed tomography (PET-CT) if no evidence of metastatic disease is present.

Barium swallow is clinically indicated if patients are suspected to be aspirating or there is concern for a tracheoesophageal fistula. Laboratory studies, including complete blood count, complete metabolic panel, liver enzymes, and nutrition-focused studies, including prealbumin for a baseline test, will be obtained. This bloodwork will help to determine if any tumor-related change to the chemistry occurs, including anemia or malnutrition.

Physical examination involves a thorough head-to-toe assessment, as patients will also be evaluated for appropriate treatments. Patients who report a decreased caloric intake require special focus on signs of dehydration and malnutrition. Any palpable lymph node may be a sign of metastatic disease, particularly Virchow node in the left supraclavicular fossa.

Endoscopic ultrasound (EUS) is performed in patients with nonmetastatic disease because it can assess the depth of local tumor invasion and any pathologic lymph nodes in the peritumoral area. EUS indicates the extent of local and regional disease and assesses the feasibility of each treatment modality, including surgical resection. Fine needle aspiration (FNA) is performed on enlarged or suspicious-appearing lymph nodes under ultrasound guidance. EUS should be performed after PET-CT of any hypermetabolically active lymph nodes to determine if a particular area should be targeted for FNA. Additionally, if endoscopy with biopsies is performed within a day or so prior to the PET, inflammation may be falsely reported as increased hypermetabolic activity in the areas examined.

Factors when discussing the use of EUS as an invasive procedure include an increased risk of aspiration, perforation, and bleeding. If stenosis or stricture of the esophagus due to tumor or other factors is present, the ultrasound probe may not be able to pass by, thus limiting its clinical utility. Unnecessary EUS should be avoided in patients who are known to have metastatic disease, as it is likely not to affect treatment or clinical outcome with an increased risk of an invasive procedure. Patients may report frustration with having to undergo an additional invasive procedure after the initial endoscopy, which likely was only performed to determine the reason for dysphagia. EUS is generally not performed unless the patient has a known diagnosis of malignancy. It is the role of the nurse and the advanced practice nurse to explain the importance of the EUS in staging and guiding the treatment plan. The utility of EUS is dependent on the experience and expertise of the endoscopist performing the procedure.

EUS plays an important role in staging, as Hulshoff et al. (2017) identified that 29% of patients who underwent EUS received treatment based on the results. EUS guides the lymph nodes that may be targeted with radiation therapy or surgically resected (Hulshoff et al., 2017). These nodes are important to identify because the rate of recurrence in regional lymph nodes after chemotherapy, radiation, and surgery is still high (Hulshoff et al., 2017).

In patients who present with dysphagia, EUS was more likely to show locally advanced disease (Mansfield, El-Dika, Krishna, Perry, & Walker, 2017). The results of this study suggest limited utility of EUS in treatment decision making and modality in patients with an obstructing mass on initial endoscopy (Mansfield et al., 2017). However, without EUS, the interprofessional team would not be able to determine if disease is present in specific lymph nodes that would benefit from resection or treatment within the radiation fields (Mansfield et al., 2017).

Clinical Staging

Accurate staging is essential to determine the correct treatment for patients and to define the goals of treatment, such as cure versus palliation. Staging is determined by the location of the tumor in the esophagus, involvement of regional lymph nodes, and presence or absence of metastatic disease (Rice, Patil, & Blackstone, 2017).

The tumor is described by its depth into the esophageal wall. T1 tumors are subdivided into T1a tumors, which invade the lamina propria or muscularis mucosae, and T1b tumors, which invade the submucosa. T2 tumors invade the muscularis propria, and T3 tumors invade the adventitia. T4 tumors invade adjacent structures. T4a tumors are considered resectable if they invade the pleura, pericardium, or diaphragm, as these structure are possible sites of tumor dissection. T4b tumors are considered unresectable, as they invade vital organs such as the aorta or trachea or structures such as the vertebral bodies. Generally, if patients have dysphagia, the tumor is usually at least T2 or T3 (Abbas & Krasna, 2017).

Regional lymph nodes are identified as suspiciously pathologic on imaging or biopsy proven via FNA. N1 disease is defined as one to two lymph nodes with metastatic disease present. N2 disease is metastasis in three to six regional lymph nodes. N3 disease is cancer seen in seven or more regional lymph nodes.

Metastasis is defined as a spread of cancer from the original site of disease to a distant organ. M1 esophageal cancer is the evidence of esophageal tumor cells in a distant organ. Special attention should be given to the liver on imaging; however, metastasis is possible anywhere in the body.

Additionally, staging can be described by the method in which disease was assessed, including clinical (*c*), which is based on imaging and physical examination; pathologic (*p*), which describes the findings on pathology; and ultrasound (*u*), when the staging is confirmed by ultrasound. When the pathology is evaluated after neoadjuvant therapy, the descriptor *yp* is used.

Treatment

Treatment for esophageal cancer includes a variety of modalities depending on the tumor's location, stage, and histology and the patient's comorbidities. Chemotherapy, radiation therapy, and surgery are mainstays, but endoluminal therapy and immunotherapy also may play a role in treatment. *Trimodality therapy* refers to the use of concurrent chemoradiation followed by surgical resection; this treatment has a curative intent. This combination of chemotherapy, radiation, and surgery occurs over a time course of about 12–16 weeks.

Chemotherapy

The goal of systemic therapy in esophageal cancer is to control tumor growth and target any micrometastasis in the lymphatics or hematogenous system (Seiwert, Salama, & Vokes, 2007). Therapy can be given with curative intent or for palliation in the setting of metastatic disease. The regimen of drugs chosen should reflect the patient's performance status, comorbid medical conditions, and toxicity profile (NCCN, 2018). Induction chemotherapy may be clinically indicated in patients with bulky disease without evidence of metastasis, as it will help to decrease the disease burden and give the disease time to declare itself if any evidence of metastasis is present. Chemotherapy can be used as a single therapy or in combination with other modalities.

For metastatic disease, systemic therapy is the primary treatment, and regimens contain two or three drugs depending on whether patients have an acceptable performance status. NCCN (2018) guidelines recommend docetaxel, cisplatin, and 5-fluorouracil (DCF); epirubicin, cisplatin, and 5-fluorouracil (ECF); or modifications with two drugs. Second-line therapy includes paclitaxel for EAC, or single-agent docetaxel, paclitaxel, or irinotecan.

Immunotherapy

Immunotherapy is designed to improve, target, or restore patients' immune function to target cancer cells (Le Bras, Farooq, Falk, & Andl, 2016). Currently, limited U.S. Food and Drug Administration–approved immunotherapy treatments are available for esophageal cancer. Ramucirumab is a monoclonal antibody that blocks vascular endothelial growth factor signaling to inhibit neoangiogenesis and is approved for advanced gastric or GEJ adenocarcinoma (Shaib, Nammour, Gill, Mody, & Saba, 2016). Trastuzumab is approved for use in patients with overexpression of HER2 in advanced esophageal cancer. Clinical trials are ongoing to detect whether esophageal cancer would be responsive to checkpoint inhibitors, including programmed cell death protein-ligand 1 (known as PD-L1) and cytotoxic T-lymphocyte antigen 4 (known as CTLA-4) inhibitors (Shaib et al., 2016). The ongoing studies bring hope to a disease with few options once it has metastasized.

HER2 gene expression has been identified in the origin of esophageal and gastric cancers. It is more commonly found in EAC than SCC and more common in GEJ than gastric (NCCN, 2018). The role of HER2 expression in relation to prognosis is not clear; however, patients with overamplification are more likely to have lymph node metastasis and extensive tumor invasion, which is correlated with poorer survival. HER2 testing is recommended for all patients with metastatic GEJ adenocarcinoma at diagnosis (NCCN, 2018). In patients with metastatic disease who have had their tumor assessed as having an overexpression of HER2, the recommended treatment is trastuzumab either as a single agent or in combination with additional chemotherapy (NCCN, 2018).

Radiation Therapy

Radiation therapy is given to reduce the risk of local recurrence and is used to treat disease in the esophagus. Radiation directly damages DNA and causes cytotoxicity, which is a benefit to targeting rapidly dividing malignant cells (Raghunathan, Khilji, Hassan, & Yusuf, 2017). When radiation is given preoperatively, the benefits include better tolerance of therapy, downstaging of the primary tumor, and enhancement of surgical resection rates (Ilson, 2017). When the tumor is resected following radiation, the pathology assessment can include the response to therapy (Ilson, 2017). Also, patients who undergo preoperative radiation will have time for the disease to declare itself as metastatic and may spare patients from an invasive surgical resection.

Radiation dosing will be based on the total intent of treatment, trimodality or bimodality. The radiation oncologist performs simulation through a specialized CT prior to the beginning of therapy to plan where the radiation will be given in the body. Careful attention is given to avoid high doses of radiation to vital structures, including the heart, lungs, and spinal cord. Patients need to be able to tolerate lying supine to be a candidate for radiation therapy. The gross tumor volume should include the primary tumor and involved lymph nodes, as well as suspicious nodes in the region of the tumor. Radiation dosing is measured in gray (Gy). Patients who are considered ineligible for surgery because of medical comorbidities or extent of disease may receive a higher radiation dose (50–50.4 Gy) to increase the chance of eradicating the disease (NCCN, 2018). Patients who are considered surgical candidates after neoadjuvant therapy will likely receive a lower dose (41.4–50.4 Gy) to preserve more of the esophageal tissue, as it will be necessary for esophageal reconstruction. The total number of fractions, or radiation sessions, would be approximately 25 to reach the total dose of therapy in the definitive or neoadjuvant setting (NCCN, 2018).

Intensity-modulated radiation therapy (IMRT) has been used to improve tumor coverage and limit normal tissue toxicities. It also allows for precise target conformity (Yang, McClosky, & Khushalani, 2009). IMRT requires the radiation oncologist to define target volumes with greater specificity (Wu et al., 2015).

Proton therapy is used in a variety of solid malignancies. It has been noted to have a sharper radiation dose falloff and less integral radiation dose compared to photon radiation (Ng & Lee, 2017). The advantages of proton therapy as opposed to traditional photon therapy are a decrease in adverse events, fewer postoperative events when surgery follows radiation, and decreased hospitalization following surgery. A review of the literature reported a comparable overall survival and local control rate when comparing proton and photon radiation treatments (Verma, Lin, Simone, & Mehta, 2016).

Concurrent Chemoradiation Therapy

In neoadjuvant treatment before surgery, the goal is for concurrent chemotherapy and radiation to eradicate the tumor or decrease tumor burden prior to surgical resection, or it can be used as a definitive treatment. Concurrent chemoradiation is a distinct treatment modality from the two techniques given separately. Chemotherapy acts as a radiosensitizer and aids the destruction of radioresistant clones and improves the chance for local control and possibly survival (Seiwert et al., 2007).

In definitive chemoradiation, therapy has a more focused organ-sparing intent, which results in improved cosmesis and function. Definitive therapy is used in patients who are not surgical candidates. Patients who were noted to be medically inoperable rather than unresectable due to the size and location of the tumor were more likely to have hospital admissions with the inability to complete the full prescribed course of concurrent chemoradiation treatment (Haj Mohammad et al., 2014). Regimens recommended by NCCN guidelines include paclitaxel and carboplatin; oxaliplatin and 5-fluorouracil; and cisplatin and 5-fluorouracil. When patients are undergoing concurrent treatment, chemotherapy is administered once a week (NCCN, 2018).

Neoadjuvant chemoradiation followed by surgical resection has been shown to have an increase in survival as compared to surgery alone. Van Hagen et al. (2012) described that 92% of patients who underwent preoperative chemoradiation had an R0 resection, meaning there were clear margins on final pathology, versus 69% of patients who underwent surgery alone. Complete pathologic response, which is no evidence of malignancy on final surgical pathology, occurred in 29% of patients who underwent chemoradiation followed by surgery. At five years, the overall survival in the chemoradiation group with surgery was 47%, as opposed to 34% for the surgery-alone group (van Hagen et al., 2012). This was also discussed in the CROSS trial, which showed an increased overall survival rate in the chemoradiation plus surgery group of 47% at five years, as opposed to 33% in the surgery-alone group (Shapiro et al., 2015). Swisher et al. (2010) reported a three-year survival rate of 29% in surgery-alone patients and 48% in patients who underwent chemoradiation and surgery.

At the completion of concurrent chemoradiation therapy, patients will undergo restaging with endoscopy and PET-CT to assess disease status. The goal of treatment is to identify a lack of residual disease on pathology and no evidence of distant metastasis on imaging; this is called a *complete clinical response*. Treatment-related changes will likely be seen on endoscopy because of radiation inflammation, and evidence of inflammation may also be present on imaging at the area of the esophagus targeted by radiation. The patient and surgeon will discuss the results and determine if surgery is appropriate. If the patient is noted to have high-risk medical comorbidities with a low-risk tumor based on pathology and disease presentation, the patient and surgeon may elect for observation. The patient would continue with a PET and endoscopy every three months to determine disease stability. Even with a complete clinical response from chemoradiation, residual disease may still be present, particularly in patients who had a large tumor or bulky adenopathy at presentation. Trials are ongoing to give better clarity on which patients would benefit more from pursuing surgery (Noordman et al., 2015).

Endoluminal Therapy

Endoluminal therapy refers to treatment only within the lumen of the esophagus. This is a minimally invasive, organ-sparing endoscopic approach to the removal of benign and early malignant tumors of the GI tract. Endoscopic mucosal resection (EMR) is reserved for smaller lesions believed to involve only the mucosa and submucosa layers (T1a and T1b lesions). An endoscopist or thoracic surgeon with appropriate training performs the procedure. Endoscopy identifies the area of confirmed or suspected malignancy, after which saline is injected underneath to raise the area away from the esophageal wall. A cap is then placed in the area around the location, breaking away the tissue. A snare attached to the end of the endoscope removes the area. The tissue is then sent to the pathologist for thorough evaluation. EMR can be a diagnostic tool for early-stage esophageal tumors because it clarifies which layer of the esophagus the tumor invades. Additionally, if the tumor is identified as invading only the lamina propria or muscularis mucosae (T1a) without evidence of lymphovascular invasion, EMR can be definitive therapy if the pathologist and endoscopist believe the tumor was adequately resected. T1b lesions are still considered high risk for metastatic disease and may require additional therapy because of the invasion of the submucosa and close proximity to the bloodstream and lymphatics. EMR for superficial SCC has been shown to have a low complication rate and a 95% five-year survival rate (Kantsevoy et al., 2008).

Surgery

Esophagectomy is the surgical resection of the esophagus, dissection of regional lymph nodes, and creation of a conduit. This is a large surgery, as it requires access to at least two body cavities: the thorax and the abdomen. Several approaches can be used, including transhiatal, Ivor

Lewis, and minimally invasive techniques with robotic assistance. Selection of surgical approach is based on tumor localization and the ability for complete resection of the tumor and its entire lymphatic drainage, which gives the best chance for long-term survival, provided the tumor can be completely removed (Seiwert et al., 2007). It is advised this procedure be performed in a high-volume center with experienced surgeons. The anatomy of the GEJ and mediastinum is complex, which increases the risk of incomplete resection and perioperative morbidity and mortality (Ilson, 2017). Esophagectomy can be offered as a stand-alone treatment in patients with early tumors (T1a, T1b, and T2) without evidence of spread to the regional lymph nodes.

Depending on the location and extent of the tumor, additional surgery may be necessary, such as for upper-third cervical tumors where a head and neck approach may be included. The conduit is generally the remaining stomach; however, the small bowel or the colon can also be used.

Preoperative evaluation includes understanding the stage of the tumor to determine if it is resectable. T4b tumors are considered unresectable because they invade essential organs. Patients with distant lymph nodes that are positive or metastatic disease in other organs are not surgical candidates, as it would be difficult to control the disease and would likely not increase survival. Patients will also undergo a thorough preoperative cardiac and pulmonary evaluation, as the surgery itself can last more than six hours. If a thoracic approach is taken, patients may require deflation of a lung during surgery. Patients with cardiac history may require cardiac clearance with stress test. Patients who are smoking close to surgery are at higher risk for postoperative complications; therefore, smoking cessation is essential.

Good communication and education are imperative to the preoperative teaching process. Preoperative teaching prepares patients for the immediate postoperative period and the life-changing issues that come after the surgery. Immediately after surgery, when patients wake from anesthesia, they will have several medical devices, including a nasogastric tube, indwelling urinary catheter, jejunostomy tube, chest tube, and IV lines. This can be alarming to patients and requires explanation. In the long term, patients will need to commit to changes in diet and sleeping habits. Patients need to understand that these changes will be lifelong; however, with proper teaching and support, it is possible to adjust to the lifestyle. Patients should be well educated on the need for commitment to lifestyle changes and the role they must play in their own recovery.

In the postoperative period, patients can expect a recovery that will include 6–10 days in the hospital and continued progress at home. Resuming normal activities can take up to 8–12 weeks, with continued adaptation to the postesophagectomy lifestyle taking up to one year. Time in the hospital has been decreased in part because of an effort to fast-track patients through the hospital experience. Patients can be safely monitored on a telemetry inpatient hospital unit with expert nursing care rather than the surgical intensive care unit (Shewale et al., 2015).

Patients will continue to remain NPO (nothing by mouth) in the immediate postoperative period because of the risk of esophageal anastomotic leak. The anastomosis is the site of the connection between the adjacent parts of the GI tract with the creation of the new conduit, where, in many cases, the surgeon has handsewn this area together. The anastomosis needs time to heal before fluids and foods can be passed through. Jejunostomy tube feedings will generally begin on postoperative day 3 after the return of bowel function has been assessed through positive bowel sounds, bowel movement, or passing of flatulence. The nasogastric tube is placed for decompression of the stomach and typically discontinued on postoperative day 5. A barium swallow to assess for anastomotic leak can be done as an outpatient procedure around postoperative day 10 or sooner depending on recovery. Patients can initiate oral intake once no evidence of leak has been identified.

Patients will have postoperative pain that requires management through a variety of regimens. Patients may require an epidural catheter for administration of pain medication. Pain management is also being developed to follow a postesophagectomy enhanced recovery after surgery (ERAS) model. With this model, medication includes local injection of bupivacaine in the surgical incisions, which serves as a nerve block to assist in the healing. Additionally, patients are prescribed anti-inflammatory medication, opioid analgesics, and gamma-aminobutyric acid analogs to decrease pain perception through multiple pathways. The ERAS model encourages a decrease in the amount of narcotics and time spent in the hospital after surgery. IV pain medication may be used in place of an epidural in the acute postoperative period and in addition to the ERAS medications. Early ambulation also is encouraged; patients will be encouraged to ambulate four hours after arrival to the inpatient hospital unit from the postanesthesia care unit. Patient will continue ambulation three to four times per day while hospitalized.

The adverse events of esophagectomy can be severe, including respiratory or cardiac failure, and the 30-day mortality for this procedure can reach up to 6% (Markar, Karthikesalingam, Thrumurthy, & Low, 2012). Patients also have continued postoperative risks, such as pneumonia, venous thromboembolism events, and postoperative infections. Adverse events specific to esophagectomy are dumping syndrome, reflux, anastomotic stricture, and gastroparesis.

Dumping syndrome is a clinical diagnosis distinguished by GI symptoms of postprandial cramping, bloating, nausea, and diarrhea and vasomotor symptoms of flushing, diaphoresis, syncope, and palpitations (Engstad & Schipper, 2009). Several interventions can mitigate the symptoms of dumping syndrome. This includes diet modification through the avoidance of high carbohydrate loads, including simple sugars. Altering traditional mealtimes to small, frequent meals, about six per day, and restricting fluid intake with meals have been shown to help the majority of patients. Fluids with meals can increase gastric motility; as such, patients should restrict fluids with meals and for 30 minutes after eating. Patients may need to avoid dairy products. Increased fiber intake has been shown to treat hypoglycemia, and proteins and fats have been shown to decrease symptoms (Berg & McCallum, 2016).

Reflux is a common postoperative change in patients who undergo esophagectomy and reconstruction because the procedure disrupts normal antireflux mechanisms through the loss of the lower esophageal sphincter. The disturbance of positive abdominal pressure and negative thoracic pressure promotes reflux as well. Patients most commonly report symptoms of pain, cough, and aspiration, with severity possibly related to the site of the anastomosis. Symptomatic patients may require the use of medical therapy such as proton pump inhibitors (PPIs) or H_2 blockers (Engstad & Schipper, 2009). Additional interventions include small, frequent feedings and elevation of patient's head while lying supine in bed to at least a 30° angle for life. This is also critical to prevent aspiration pneumonia. Avoiding meals three hours before bed will also limit the amount of reflux.

Esophageal anastomotic stricture is one of the most common complications after esophagectomy, with an incidence of 10%–40%. Symptoms include dysphagia and postprandial fullness (Huang et al., 2015). Esophageal stricture typically develops two to six months after surgery and may be due to tension and inadequate blood supply (Engstad & Schipper, 2009). Higher rates have been reported in patients who had a complication of anastomotic leak after surgery (Gamliel & Krasna, 2009). Patients may relate swallowing problems to recurrence of cancer and become very alarmed at the development of these symptoms (Tsottles, Lang, & Choflet, 2018). Evaluation for esophageal stricture includes barium swallow, EUS, and chest CT (Argote-Greene & Sugarbaker, 2009). Postoperative dysphagia should be evaluated with endoscopic or radiographic confirmation, as one-third of patients with dysphagia will not have stricture (Engstad & Schipper, 2009). The intervention for esophageal stricture includes dilation, which involves expansible forces against a luminal stenosis. Bougie dilators or balloon dilators can be used for stenosis through an endoscopic procedure using a dilator and guidewire (Siddiqui et al., 2013). Treatment with endoscopic dilation is successful in 80%–90% of patients; however, some patients may need to undergo dilation every two to three weeks until a complete response occurs (van Boeckel & Siersema, 2015). Steroid injection or self-dilation at home can also be attempted in patients with refractory stricture.

Gastroparesis is defined as objectively delayed gastric emptying in the absence of mechanical obstruction (Camilleri, Parkman, Shafi, Abell, & Gerson, 2013). Clinical manifestations are noted in 10%–50% of patients after esophagectomy (Argote-Greene & Sugarbaker, 2009). Symptoms of gastroparesis include nausea, vomiting, early satiety, and epigastric pain. Gastroparesis can be caused early in the postoperative period by edema in the mucosa and generally resolves in 10–14 days (Battafarano & Patterson, 2008). Treatment focuses on symptom management, including dietary changes, and ensuring that patients follow the postesophagectomy diet, including eating small, frequent meals as opposed to three large meals. Patients with gastroparesis should avoid high-fat foods and high-fiber foods because they decrease gastric motility (Fogle, 2013). Gastroparesis can be treated with pyloric dilation after surgery. Botulinum toxin (Botox®) injection intraoperatively has been noted to decrease gastroparesis in the postoperative period (Akkerman, Haverkamp, van Hillegersberg, & Ruurda, 2014; see Table 2-2).

Palliation

Palliative therapy includes treatment of symptoms when the goal of treatment is not cure but rather comfort in patients with a tumor that

Table 2-2. Interventions for Adverse Effects of Esophagectomy

Adverse Effect	Symptoms	Interventions
Dumping syndrome	Bloating, diaphoresis, diarrhea, flushing, nausea, palpitations, postprandial cramping, syncope	Diet modification; small, frequent meals; medication
Esophageal stricture	Dysphagia, postprandial fullness	Dilation via upper endoscopy, self-dilation, steroid injections
Gastroparesis	Early satiety, epigastric pain, nausea, vomiting	Diet modification, prokinetic medication to promote gastric motility
Reflux	Aspiration, cough, pain	Elevation of the head of the bed to 30° when supine; medical therapy; small, frequent meals

Note. Based on information from Akkerman et al., 2014; Berg & McCallum, 2016; Engstad & Schipper, 2009; Siddiqui et al., 2013.

has advanced. Additionally, patients may require palliative measures before the tumor is treated locally if it is causing significant dysphagia or pain. In regard to dysphagia, patients may require an esophageal stent to be placed at the site of the tumor, which would allow for the passage of food and liquids through the esophagus. Stents can also be used in patients who develop significant stricture related to prior radiation therapy or surgery. Argon-plasma coagulation, photodynamic therapy, and brachytherapy are local therapies in the esophagus to control the tumor and allow for relief of dysphagia (Rabenstein, 2015). Esophageal stent placement provides more immediate relief as compared to external radiation or brachytherapy. This may be preferred in patients who are symptomatic and have a limited expected survival.

Bleeding can occur at the site of the tumor. Cauterization, clipping, or injection of medication may be required to stop the bleeding. Palliative radiation can be given to areas causing pain in metastatic sites. Patients who present or progress to stage IV disease should have an early referral to palliative care for assistance in symptom management, including pain and nausea or vomiting. Esophageal cancer is highly symptomatic, and not addressing these needs early can lead to increased patient stress and anxiety.

Nursing Care

Patients who receive chemotherapy must have adequate IV access. Nursing assessment includes the ability of the veins to tolerate the administration of vesicants and irritants. Nurses may have to advocate for a central line, such as a port, to be placed for safe administration.

Antiemetic regimens for patients undergoing chemotherapy include assessment of the emetogenic propensity of the drugs. The best way to control nausea and vomiting is to prevent them before they start. Several of the regimens for esophageal cancer contain cisplatin, which has a high potential to cause emesis. Patients may require premedication with IV administration of a $5-HT_3$ receptor antagonist and a corticosteroid. Antinausea medication may be continued for several days after the infusion. Patients will also receive a prescription to take orally as needed for nausea. Patients undergoing chemotherapy may also complain of taste changes that can lead to nausea; thus, patients should eat a variety of foods and determine the ones that are most palatable.

Nursing care with radiation therapy rests largely on educating and supporting patients through treatment. Dermatitis is a risk whenever radiation is given. Patients can use moisturizer prophylactically to prevent severe reactions (Fogh & Yom, 2014). Radiation pneumonitis occurs typically one to three months after completion of radiation to the thorax. Patients can present with respiratory symptoms, including cough, shortness of breath, and pleuritic chest pain with a low-grade fever, and can progress to severe symptoms, including respiratory failure. Evidence is seen radiographically as opacities in the lungs that are not explained by pneumonia or pleural effusion. Treatment includes steroids to decrease this altered immune response. Fatigue is a distressing factor for patients and can become acutely apparent during radiation therapy. Sleep hygiene should be stressed before medical therapy is attempted (Fogh & Yom, 2014).

When discussing the adverse events and side effects of radiation to the esophagus, an important one to highlight is radiation esophagitis. As opposed to radiation to the thorax for other cancers to the chest, including breast and lung, treatment will not spare the esophagus from a full treatment dose. Patients are much more likely to experience some degree of esophagitis. It has been reported that patients who receive concurrent chemotherapy and radiation are at a higher risk for esophagitis than those receiving radiation alone (Fogh & Yom, 2014). Patients will require appropriate pain management, which may include topical opioid medication including liquid morphine. It is not uncommon for patients to require enteral tube feeding during radiation to maintain adequate caloric intake and hydration. Genetic variations may influence inflammatory reactions that can increase patients' propensity to have a more severe form of radiation esophagitis (Murro & Jakate, 2015).

Nutrition

Nurses will document an accurate assessment of what patients are taking in for calories, or calorie counts. This will allow for an understanding of patients' baseline and actual nutritional needs. The patient's height and weight will need to be accurately documented to determine true body mass index. Patients undergoing chemotherapy may have a changed palate, and nurses can encourage them to try a variety of high-calorie and high-protein foods and supplements.

Patients who have undergone esophagectomy will need teaching and encouragement on eating six smaller meals a day with decreased intake of simple carbohydrates to avoid dumping syndrome. Patients often have many questions about what foods are appropriate. Consultation with a registered dietitian is important to guide patients through this process.

Enteral Tube Feeding

Patients who require enteral tube feedings cannot maintain an adequate nutrient level through oral intake. For patients with esophageal cancer, several reasons may cause this, including the location of the tumor itself, which may prohibit the passage of food; healing from surgery, which may cause patients to be NPO for a period of time; or complications from radiation esophagitis. Assessment will also include skin integrity, as patients with poor nutrition are at high risk for skin breakdown.

A gastrostomy tube, or prepyloric tube, can be used in patients who will not have surgery involving the stomach. A gastrostomy tube allows for absorption of medications and nutrients from the stomach. A jejunostomy tube, or postpyloric tube, can also be used depending on the location of the tumor and the planned surgical resection. Nurses caring for patients with an enteral feeding tube will teach patients and families how to care for the tube at home. Patients will also use the tube for the administration of medication, as dysphagia may prohibit taking medications by the standard route. This requires collaboration with the pharmacy and physician to ensure that patients can obtain all necessary medications.

Nurses are advocates for patients in this setting, as the nursing assessment may reveal malnourishment and other factors that may lead to patients being unable to obtain proper intake of food. Consulting with a registered dietitian is also crucial to ensure that patients are on the proper formula and receiving the correct number of calories. Patients and family members will need instruction on how to clean the tube with water. Nurses also will assess for skin infections at the site of the tube. The tube may have a plastic disc that sits flush against the skin, and some tubes are sutured in place. If the tube were to dislodge partway, patients should be instructed to reinsert the portion of the tube that has come out and secure it to the abdominal wall with tape. If the tube completely dislodges, patients are to cover the area and report to the emergency department for reinsertion of the tube.

Nursing assessment for patients with a tube in place also includes evaluating for abdominal distension, rigidity, and residual in the GI tract to assess for absorption. It will be necessary to auscultate for bowel sounds. Thorough assessment includes discussing bowel movements with patients, as they may be more prone to diarrhea. This may be able to be adjusted with a change in formula or addition of fiber. Communication and consultation with a dietitian should remain open.

Physical Activity

Patients undergoing cancer treatment often suffer from fatigue and treatment-related changes to physical stamina. Patients undergoing neoadjuvant chemoradiation who were assigned to a three-times-a-week walking program led by a nurse and a weekly nutritional support group had better outcomes compared to patients who did not undergo these interventions (Xu et al., 2015). Patients in the intervention group were able to maintain their physical endurance, muscle strength, and weight better than those in the control group. This information can be used to encourage patients to remain physically active and maintain nutritional goals during therapy. This will also help to counteract some symptoms of fatigue.

Communication

Patients with esophageal cancer will have many questions and concerns because of the nature of the disease and the complexity of the treatment. Patients who completed treatment reported the support of the clinical nurse specialist was important throughout treatment and recovery. Patients also described they often needed clarification to understand the disease process and the treatment plan and looked to their nurse for this support (Graham & Wikman, 2016). Weekly nursing phone calls to patients at home after surgery were found to increase patient satisfaction with understanding of information (Malmström et al., 2016).

Esophageal cancer is noted to have one of the highest rates of suicide when compared to other malignancies. Patients are more likely to commit suicide in the first 12 weeks after diagnosis (Graham & Wikman, 2016). Nurses should perform distress scale assessments at baseline and as needed to uncover any psychosocial issues that may be related to the recent diagnosis or the continued adjustment during treatment and recovery. Referral to psychiatry and counseling should be made as appropriate.

Prognosis

The prognosis of esophageal cancer remains poor for the total diagnosed. The majority of patients present with metastatic disease in which cure is not possible. For all stages of disease, the five-year survival rate is 19.2%, according to data from the Surveillance, Epidemiology, and End Results (SEER) Program (n.d.). Strides have been made in early- and regional-stage diseases, as patients with early-stage disease treated with EMR have a 95% survival rate at five years (Kantsevoy et al., 2008). Local-regional disease with spread to lymph nodes is noted to have improved prognosis with the use of neoadjuvant chemoradiation. Much progress remains to be made; however, management and treatment options have improved in the past 40 years, as the five-year survival rate was 4% in 1975 according to SEER data (SEER Program, n.d.).

Prevention

Esophageal cancer has a number of risk factors that can be modified to decrease the incidence. EAC has been directly linked to BE through the complications of GERD. Prevention of the progression of metaplasia to dysplasia to adenocarcinoma will help to decrease the rate of EAC in these patients. Procedures with radiofrequency ablation and EMR are used to ensure the eradication of metaplasia. With the addition of PPI therapy twice a day, 93% of patients achieved complete eradication of intestinal metaplasia (Komanduri et al., 2017).

PPIs are used for patients with GERD, BE, and chronic use of nonsteroidal anti-inflammatory drugs (NSAIDs) to decrease the amount of acid being produced and to protect the epithelium of the stomach and the esophagus. Retrospective reports have linked long-term use to multiple adverse events, including kidney disease, dementia, diminished bone density, micronutrient deficiencies, and infections, particularly in the gut. These are all thought to be the result of functional acid suppression caused by the PPIs. The majority of these claims have been made after retrospective review of the evidence, and it is therefore difficult to extrapolate the results (Freedberg, Kim, & Yang, 2017). Freedberg et al. (2017) stated that the long-term use of PPIs in patients for whom it is appropriate is likely to be more beneficial than harmful.

Smoking tobacco has been directly linked to SCC and EAC. Smoking cessation and abstinence is important to decrease the risk of esophageal cancer. Excessive alcohol intake has been directly linked to SCC of the esophagus. The American Cancer Society recommends a maximum of one alcoholic beverage a day for women and two per day for men as a guideline to alcohol intake for cancer prevention (Kushi et al., 2012).

Epidemiologic evidence has suggested that aspirin and NSAIDs are related to a decrease in esophageal cancer. This has not been proved, and evidence is insufficient to recommend wide use, as prolonged use of NSAIDs and aspirin in combination produces side effects (Zakko et al., 2017).

Obesity is known to cause inflammation in the body and produce hormones that may contribute to the development of cancer. Increased pressure in the abdomen due to central adiposity related to obesity has been correlated to the development of EAC. Encouraging patients to maintain a healthy weight would help to decrease this risk (Abbas & Krasna, 2017).

No current guidelines exist for esophageal cancer screening in the United States. The American College of Gastroenterology recommends screening for BE in men with chronic reflux and other risk factors every three to five years (Griffin-Sobel, 2017). The National Cancer Institute (2018) reported that routine screening would result in no or minimal decrease in mortality from esophageal cancer in the U.S. population. The harm associated with screening would include serious but uncommon adverse events related to endoscopy, including esophageal perforation, aspiration, and bleeding that necessitates hospitalization. It is again important to highlight that patients who have BE have an increased risk of cancer but that it is still a very low risk overall. Patients with BE may incur psychological harm by believing they are at a very high risk for developing cancer.

High-Risk Assessment: Screening and Genetic Testing

Currently, few identified inherited genes are directly linked to the development of esophageal cancer. Patients with Fanconi anemia, which is a rare recessive genetic syndrome, are noted to be at an increased risk of several cancers, including esophageal. Patients with a family history of oral or pharyngeal cancer were noted to be at a higher risk for esophageal cancer in case-control studies. Patients with cancer genetic syndromes such as Li-Fraumeni syndrome may be at higher risk for esophageal cancer (Turati, Negri, & La Vecchia, 2014). Bloom syndrome has been associated with an increased risk of esophageal cancer, and screening for GERD symptoms at the age of 20 with or without endoscopy may be considered. Patients with nonepidermolytic palmoplantar keratosis and Howel-Evans syndrome are also candidates for screening with endoscopy after the age of 20 because of the increased risk of esophageal cancer (NCCN, 2018).

Increased interest lies in identifying patients with BE who may progress to EAC and how to determine these high-risk patients. *Microsatellite instability* describes the loss of heterozygosity and the emergence of new alleles, which leads to dysplasia and BE. The extent of genomic instability, measured as a mutational load in a biopsy of BE, can predict the risk of progression to adenocarcinoma in patients who would have otherwise been deemed low risk based on histologic findings alone (Abbas & Krasna, 2017). These techniques are currently being investigated. It is cautioned that patients may be overdiagnosed and undergo unnecessary testing and treatment. Additionally, other patients may be underdiagnosed, leading to not being appropriately treated, which can lead to EAC (Reid, 2017).

Microsatellite instability is also tested in patients with metastatic disease. Pembrolizumab has been approved for patients with microsatellite instability–high disease. It is recommended that all patients with unresectable or metastatic EAC disease be tested for microsatellite instability (NCCN, 2018).

Surveillance

Follow-up per NCCN (2018) guidelines for patients who underwent treatment for esophageal cancer includes screening for recurrence of disease and side effect management. Asymptomatic patients should undergo a complete history and physical every 3–6 months for 1–2 years, then every 6–12 months for 3–5 years, and annually thereafter. This surveillance will also include imaging studies, endoscopy with biopsy, and blood work depending on clinical necessity and symptoms (NCCN, 2018).

Survivorship

Cancer survivorship is defined in a variety of paradigms, including from the moment of diagnosis. Particular interest is focused on patients with esophageal cancer who undergo extensive treatments and invasive procedures related to quality of life. For patients with regional disease, the recommended therapy may include two or three treatments with long-term side effects requiring particular nursing assessment and support as they move from active treatment to the surveillance phase of the cancer trajectory. Cancer survivors report an overall poorer quality of life when compared to the general population because of the adverse effects of therapy and anxiety of recurrence (Jefford et al., 2017). Survival rates and durable time without disease are increasing, thus making survivorship care plans and understanding of long-term side effects of more interest to researchers.

Quality of life for survivors who underwent esophagectomy has been heavily researched and discussed in the literature. It should be acknowledged as a subjective measure, as it is patient reported based on individual experiences. Patients will go through a response shift as their perceptions change over time and they adjust to their new normal (Darling, 2013). Symptom management assessment should be detailed in this population and specific to the cancer and the esophagectomy symptoms (Ginex et al., 2013). At one year postoperatively, patients still frequently noted lack of energy, feeling full too quickly, drowsiness, and difficulty sleeping. At six months, patients reported significant symptoms. However, by 12 months, the symptoms lessened and were comparable to preoperative levels. In a meta-analysis comparing health-related quality of life in patients who underwent minimally invasive esophagectomy versus open esophagectomy, the researchers noted better outcomes in regard to symptoms at three months in the minimally invasive group. However, these differences were not detected at 6 and 12 months (Kauppila, Xie, Johar, Markar, & Lagergren, 2017).

Quality of life following esophagectomy when assessed in comparison to long-term follow-up has similar results to the general population (Darling, 2013). Quality of life five years after esophagectomy has been described at levels equal to the background population. This lends to the idea that patients who do report poor quality of life may need supportive interventions sooner (Derogar & Lagergren, 2012). Conflicting evidence has been reported in evaluation of the long-term follow-up of survivors after more than 10 years. Schandl, Lagergren, Johar, and Lagergren (2016) described significant deterioration in quality of life, role functioning, social functioning, and symptoms including reflux, diarrhea, and weight loss among patients who survived more than 10 years. Greene et al. (2014) described that in the majority of patients who survived an average of 12 years, most had no dysphagia and were able to comfortably eat with few symptoms of dumping syndrome or reflux.

Esophagectomy is known to have a significant negative effect on physical fitness and health-related quality of life (Greene et al., 2014). In qualitative research, patients who have undergone esophagectomy have described the procedure as "remapping the body" (Wainwright, Donovan, Kavadas, Cramer, & Blazeby, 2007, p. 760). Additionally, these patients have described changes to swallowing and taste that made eating less pleasurable and required much organization and planning. Patients who undergo any treatment for esophageal cancer may have body image concerns about losing weight and the feeding tube looking bunchy underneath their clothes. Social changes also occur, as difficulty swallowing and feeding tubes take away from the normalcy of sitting down and eating a meal with loved ones, which may lead to isolation.

Patients who undergo thoracic radiation are noted to be at an increased risk for cardiovascular disease many years after the completion of treatment. Radiation to the thorax and mediastinum is correlated with an early onset of coronary artery disease 5–20 years after the completion of therapy in cancer survivors, even in the absence of other risk factors. Radiation techniques have become more precise in eradicating cancer with longer survival. However, patients are living longer to experience these distant side effects. When working with long-term survivors of esophageal cancer, healthcare providers should assess for history of radiation therapy to help determine if additional assessment should be given to include cardiovascular screening. No current guidelines exist for the interval or recommendation for this issue (Raghunathan et al., 2017).

Patients who undergo esophagectomy are noted to have nutritional deficits, including vitamin deficiencies and sustained weight loss with loss of muscle mass. In a study of 66 patients, 73% had evidence of malabsorption related to radiation changes that affected the pancreas and postoperative changes. Intervention may include supplementation of pancreatic enzymes and other vitamins. Additional research is still needed in this area to apply clinical changes that would be meaningful to patients (Heneghan et al., 2015).

Comparison of Esophageal and Gastric Cancers

Esophageal and gastric cancers are tumors of the upper GI tract. They may present with similarities but are treated differently based on the pathology, location, and nature of the disease. The majority of cases present late in the disease course: half of esophageal tumors and 65% of gastric tumors present with locally advanced or metastatic disease at the time of diagnosis (Hayes, Smyth, Riddell, & Allum, 2017). Cancers of the upper GI tract are not common in the United States and are not screened for on a routine basis (NCCN, 2018).

Staging for esophageal and gastric cancer regardless of the histology or location is defined using the tumor-node-metastasis, or TNM, staging system, which assigns a stage of I to IV (Hayes et al., 2017). Tumor stage (T) is described by the depth of invasion of the tumor into the esophageal or gastric wall. The node stage (N) is determined by the extent of lymph node metastasis in relation to the location of the tumor. For esophageal tumors, spread of lymphatic disease outside of the nodal basin, or beyond regional lymph nodes in gastric cancer, is considered metastatic disease (M), including spread to distant organs (Hayes et al., 2017).

Interprofessional team management is essential for patients with esophageal and gastric cancers (NCCN, 2018). Treatment can involve multiple modalities for both cancers and requires communication and assessment among nursing and other practitioners. The next chapter will discuss gastric cancers as separate entities, including the risk factors, symptoms, staging, treatment, and nursing care. Some similarities exist, but it is imperative to distinguish the two as distinct disease processes to tailor patient care. Nursing care related to the administration of treatment and the management of side effects may be interchangeable in some cases, but nurses need to understand the cause of symptoms in each patient.

The Siewert classification identifies the location from which the tumor arises and defines how the tumor will be treated (Siewert, Stein, & Feith, 2006). The stomach and esophagus are anatomically located close together. However, a distinction exists between the two based on the cellular and anatomic level, as the function of each organ is defined by the structure, glands, and musculature. The GEJ is defined as the anatomic distinction between the esophagus and the stomach. Histologic findings also can correlate this distinction (Siewert et al., 2006). Siewert et al. (2006) defined tumors based on location to delineate the approach for treatment. Type I tumors arise 1–5 cm proximal to the GEJ and are considered tumors of the lower esophagus; these are treated as esophageal tumors. Type II tumors arise from 1 cm proximal and 2 cm distal to the GEJ and represent cardia carcinomas; these are also treated as esophageal tumors. Type III tumors arise from 2–5 cm distal to the GEJ and are considered to be subcarinal gastric carcinomas; these are treated as gastric tumors (see Table 2-3).

Table 2-3. Siewert Classification

Type	Location at Gastroesophageal Junction	Treatment
I	1–5 cm above	Treated as esophageal tumor
II	1 cm above and 2 cm below	Treated as esophageal tumor
III	2–5 cm below	Treated as gastric tumor

Note. Based on information from Siewert et al., 2006.

Debate and controversy often arise as to how patients should be treated based on presentation in the GEJ and pathologic factors. Ultimately, the healthcare team will make the decision for therapy—to treat as an esophageal or gastric tumor—based on their belief as to what will best control the tumor (NCCN, 2018). This is a point of discussion for the interprofessional team and may require input from experts in both esophageal and gastric cancer to determine the appropriate treatment. For more information on gastric cancers, see Chapter 3.

Summary

Although still relatively rare, esophageal cancer is a disease with a rising incidence in the United States. Treatment in the curative setting can possibly involve several modalities; however, the vast majority of patients present with late-stage disease. Medicine and nursing need specialty skills to appropriately treat and manage the symptoms of this disease.

Moving forward, research is needed in additional treatments to increase the survival and the management of long-term adverse effects.

References

Abbas, G., & Krasna, M. (2017). Overview of esophageal cancer. *Annals of Cardiothoracic Surgery, 6,* 131–136. https://doi.org/10.21037/acs.2017.03.03

Akkerman, R.D.L., Haverkamp, L., van Hillegersberg, R., & Ruurda, J.P. (2014). Surgical techniques to prevent delayed gastric emptying after esophagectomy with gastric interposition: A systematic review. *Annals of Thoracic Surgery, 98,* 1512–1519. https://doi.org/10.1016/j.athoracsur.2014.06.057

American Cancer Society. (2018). *Cancer facts and figures 2018.* Atlanta, GA: Author.

Argote-Greene, L.M., & Sugarbaker, D.J. (2009). Three-hole esophagectomy: The Brigham and Women's Hospital approach. In D.J. Sugarbaker, R. Bueno, M.J. Krasna, S.J. Mentzer, & L. Zellos (Eds.), *Adult chest surgery* (pp. 141–154). New York, NY: McGraw-Hill Medical.

Battafarano, R.J., & Patterson, G.A. (2008). Complications of esophageal resection. In G.A. Patterson, J.D. Cooper, J. Deslauriers, A.E.M.R. Lerut, J.D. Luketich, & T.W. Rice (Eds.), *Pearson's thoracic and esophageal surgery* (3rd ed., pp. 545–552). Philadelphia, PA: Elsevier Churchill Livingstone.

Berg, P., & McCallum, R. (2016). Dumping syndrome: A review of the current concepts of pathophysiology, diagnosis, and treatment. *Digestive Diseases and Sciences, 61,* 11–18. https://doi.org/10.1007/s10620-015-3839-x

Camilleri, M., Parkman, H.P., Shafi, M.A., Abell, T.L., & Gerson, L. (2013). Clinical guideline: Management of gastroparesis. *American Journal of Gastroenterology, 108,* 18–37. https://doi.org/10.1038/ajg.2012.373

Darling, G.E. (2013). Quality of life in patients with esophageal cancer. *Thoracic Surgery Clinics, 23,* 569–575. https://doi.org/10.1016/j.thorsurg.2013.07.011

Derogar, M., & Lagergren, P. (2012). Health-related quality of life among 5-year survivors of esophageal cancer surgery: A prospective population-based study. *Journal of Clinical Oncology, 30,* 413–418. https://doi.org/10.1200/JCO.2011.38.9791

Engstad, K., & Schipper, P.H. (2009). Postoperative care and management of the complication of surgical therapy. In B.A. Jobe, J.G. Hunter, & C.R. Thomas Jr. (Eds.), *Esophageal cancer: Principles and practice* (pp. 659–680). New York, NY: Demos Medical.

Fogh, S., & Yom, S.S. (2014). Symptom management during the radiation oncology treatment course: A practical guide for the oncology clinician. *Seminars in Oncology, 41,* 764–775. https://doi.org/10.1053/j.seminoncol.2014.09.020

Fogle, C.J. (2013). Diabetic gastroparesis: An overview of diagnostic and treatment strategies. *Advance for NPs and PAs, 4,* 14–18.

Freedberg, D.E., Kim, L.S., & Yang, Y.-X. (2017). The risks and benefits of long-term use of proton pump inhibitors: Expert review and best practice advice from the American Gastroenterological Association. *Gastroenterology, 152,* 706–715. https://doi.org/10.1053/j.gastro.2017.01.031

Gamliel, Z., & Krasna, M. (2009). Transhiatal esophagectomy. In D.J. Sugarbaker, R. Bueno, M.J. Krasna, S.J. Mentzer, & L. Zellos (Eds.), *Adult chest surgery* (pp. 131–140). New York, NY: McGraw-Hill Medical.

Ginex, P., Thom, B., Jingeleski, M., Vincent, A., Plourde, G., Rizk, N., ... Bains, M. (2013). Patterns of symptoms following surgery for esophageal cancer [Online exclusive]. *Oncology Nursing Forum, 40,* E101–E107. https://doi.org/10.1188/13.ONF.E101-E107

Graham, L., & Wikman, A. (2016). Toward improved survivorship: Supportive care needs of esophageal cancer patients, a literature review. *Diseases of the Esophagus, 29,* 1081–1089. https://doi.org/10.1111/dote.12424

Greene, C.L., DeMeester, S.R., Worrell, S.G., Oh, D.S., Hagen, J.A., & DeMeester, T.R. (2014). Alimentary satisfaction, gastrointestinal symptoms, and quality of life 10 or more years after esophagectomy with gastric pull-up. *Journal of Thoracic and Cardiovascular Surgery, 147,* 909–914. https://doi.org/10.1016/j.jtcvs.2013.11.004

Griffin-Sobel, J.P. (2017). Gastrointestinal cancers: Screening and early detection. *Seminars in Oncology Nursing, 33,* 165–171. https://doi.org/10.1016/j.soncn.2017.02.004

Haj Mohammad, N., Hulshof, M.C., Bergman, J.J., Geijsen, D., Wilmink, J.W., van Berge Henegouwen, M.I., ... van Laarhoven, H.W. (2014). Acute toxicity of definitive chemoradiation in patients with inoperable or irresectable esophageal carcinoma. *BMC Cancer, 14,* 56. https://doi.org/10.1186/1471-2407-14-56

Hayes, T., Smyth, E., Riddell, A., & Allum, W. (2017). Staging in esophageal and gastric cancers. *Hematology/Oncology Clinics of North America, 31,* 427–440. https://doi.org/10.1016/j.hoc.2017.02.002

Heneghan, H.M., Zaborowski, A., Fanning, M., McHugh, A., Doyle, S., Moore, J., ... Reynolds, J.V. (2015). Prospective study of malabsorption and malnutrition after esophageal and gastric cancer surgery. *Annals of Surgery, 262,* 803–807. https://doi.org/10.1097/SLA.0000000000001445

Huang, Q., Zhong, J., Yang, T., Li, J., Luo, K., Zheng, Y., ... Fu, J. (2015). Impacts of anastomotic complications on the health-related quality of life after esophagectomy. *Journal of Surgical Oncology, 111,* 365–370. https://doi.org/10.1002/jso.23837

Hulshoff, J.B., Mul, V.E.M., de Boer, H.E.M., Noordzij, W., Korteweg, T., van Dullemen, H.M., ... Plukker, J.T.M. (2017). Impact of endoscopic ultrasonography on ^{18}F-FDG-PET/CT upfront towards patient specific esophageal cancer treatment. *Annals of Surgical Oncology, 24,* 1828–1834. https://doi.org/10.1245/s10434-017-5835-1

Ilson, D.H. (2017). The role of radiation therapy in upper gastrointestinal cancers. *Clinical Advances in Hematology and Oncology, 15,* 366–376.

Jefford, M., Ward, A.C., Lisy, K., Lacey, K., Emery, J.D., Glaser, A.W., ... Bishop, J. (2017). Patient-reported outcomes in cancer survivors: A population-wide cross-sectional study. *Supportive Care in Cancer, 25,* 3171–3179. https://doi.org/10.1007/s00520-017-3725-5

Kantsevoy, S.V., Adler, D.G., Conway, J.D., Diehl, D.L., Farraye, F.A., Kwon, R., ... Tierney, W.M. (2008). Endoscopic mucosal resection and endoscopic submucosal dissection. *Gastrointestinal Endoscopy, 68,* 11–18. https://doi.org/10.1016/j.gie.2008.01.037

Kauppila, J.H., Xie, S., Johar, A., Markar, S.R., & Lagergren, P. (2017). Meta-analysis of health-related quality of life after minimally invasive versus open oesophagectomy for oesophageal cancer. *British Journal of Surgery, 104,* 1131–1140. https://doi.org/10.1002/bjs.10577

Kethman, W., & Hawn, M. (2017). New approaches to gastroesophageal reflux disease. *Journal of Gastrointestinal Surgery, 21,* 1544–1552. https://doi.org/10.1007/s11605-017-3439-5

Komanduri, S., Kahrilas, P.J., Krishnan, K., McGorisk, T., Bidari, K., Grande, D., ... Pandolfino, J. (2017). Recurrence of Barrett's esophagus is rare following endoscopic eradication therapy coupled with effective reflux control. *American Journal of Gastroenterology, 112,* 556–566. https://doi.org/10.1038/ajg.2017.13

Kushi, L.H., Doyle, C., McCullough, M., Rock, C.L., Demark-Wahnefried, W., Bandera, E.V., ... Gansler, T. (2012). American Cancer Society guidelines on nutrition and physical activity for cancer prevention: Reducing the risk of cancer with healthy food choices and physical activity. *CA: A Cancer Journal for Clinicians, 62,* 30–67. https://doi.org/10.3322/caac.20140

Le Bras, G.F., Farooq, M.H., Falk, G.W., & Andl, C.D. (2016). Esophageal cancer: The latest on chemoprevention and state of the art therapies. *Pharmacology Research, 113*, 236–244. https://doi.org/10.1016/j.phrs.2016.08.021

Malhotra, G.K., Yanala, U., Ravipati, A., Follet, M., Vijayakumar, M., & Are, C. (2017). Global trends in esophageal cancer. *Journal of Surgical Oncology, 115*, 564–579. https://doi.org/10.1002/jso.24592

Malmström, M., Ivarsson, B., Klefsgård, R., Persson, K., Jakobsson, U., & Johansson, J. (2016). The effect of a nurse led telephone supportive care programme on patients' quality of life, received information and health care contacts after oesophageal cancer surgery—A six month RCT-follow-up study. *International Journal of Nursing Studies, 64*, 86–95. https://doi.org/10.1016/j.ijnurstu.2016.09.009

Mansfield, S.A., El-Dika, S., Krishna, S.G., Perry, K.A., & Walker, J.P. (2017). Routine staging with endoscopic ultrasound in patients with obstructing esophageal cancer and dysphagia rarely impacts treatment decisions. *Surgical Endoscopy, 31*, 3227–3233. https://doi.org/10.1007/s00464-016-5351-6

Markar, S.R., Karthikesalingam, A., Thrumurthy, S., & Low, D.E. (2012). Volume-outcome relationship in surgery for esophageal malignancy: Systematic review and meta-analysis 2000-2011. *Journal of Gastrointestinal Surgery, 16*, 1055–1063. https://doi.org/10.1007/s11605-011-1731-3

Morton, L.M., Gilbert, E.S., Stovall, M., van Leeuwen, F.E., Dores, G.M., Lynch, C.F., … Curtis, R.E. (2014). Risk of esophageal cancer following radiotherapy for Hodgkin lymphoma. *Haematologica, 99*, e193–e196. https://doi.org/10.3324/haematol.2014.108258

Murro, D., & Jakate, S. (2015). Radiation esophagitis. *Archives of Pathology and Laboratory Medicine, 139*, 827–830. https://doi.org/10.5858/arpa.2014-0111-RS

National Cancer Institute. (2018). Esophageal cancer screening (PDQ®) [Health professional version]. Retrieved from https://www.cancer.gov/types/esophageal/hp/esophageal-screening-pdq

National Comprehensive Cancer Network. (2018). *NCCN Clinical Practice Guidelines in Oncology (NCCN Guidelines®): Esophageal and esophagogastric junction cancers* [v.2.2018]. Retrieved from https://www.nccn.org/professionals/physician_gls/pdf/esophageal.pdf

Ng, J., & Lee, P. (2017). The role of radiotherapy in localized esophageal and gastric cancer. *Hematology/Oncology Clinics of North America, 31*, 453–468. https://doi.org/10.1016/j.hoc.2017.01.005

Noordman, B.J., Shapiro, J., Spaander, M.C., Krishnadath, K.K., van Laarhoven, H.W., van Berge Henegouwen, M.I., … van Lanschot, J.J. (2015). Accuracy of detecting residual disease after cross neoadjuvant chemoradiotherapy for esophageal cancer (preSANO Trial): Rationale and protocol. *JMIR Research Protocols, 4*, e79. https://doi.org/10.2196/resprot.4320

Oezcelik, A., & DeMeester, S.R. (2011). General anatomy of the esophagus. *Thoracic Surgery Clinics, 21*, 289–297. https://doi.org/10.1016/j.thorsurg.2011.01.003

Rabenstein, T. (2015). Palliative endoscopic therapy of esophageal cancer. *Viszeralmedizin, 31*, 354–359. https://doi.org/10.1159/000441175

Raghunathan, D., Khilji, M.I., Hassan, S.A., & Yusuf, S.W. (2017). Radiation-induced cardiovascular disease. *Current Atherosclerosis Reports, 19*, 22. https://doi.org/10.1007/s11883-017-0658-x

Reid, B.J. (2017). Genomics, endoscopy, and control of gastroesophageal cancers: A perspective. *Cellular and Molecular Gastroenterology and Hepatology, 3*, 359–366. https://doi.org/10.1016/j.jcmgh.2017.02.005

Rice, T.W., & Bronner, M.P. (2011). The esophageal wall. *Thoracic Surgery Clinics, 21*, 299–305. https://doi.org/10.1016/j.thorsurg.2011.01.005

Rice, T.W., Patil, D.T., & Blackstone, E.H. (2017). 8th edition AJCC/UICC staging of cancers of the esophagus and esophagogastric junction: Application to clinical practice. *Annals of Cardiothoracic Surgery, 6,* 119–130. https://doi.org/10.21037/acs.2017.03.14

Schandl, A., Lagergren, J., Johar, A., & Lagergren, P. (2016). Health-related quality of life 10 years after oesophageal cancer surgery. *European Journal of Cancer, 69,* 43–50. https://doi.org/10.1016/j.ejca.2016.09.032

Seiwert, T.Y., Salama, J.K., & Vokes, E.E. (2007). The concurrent chemoradiation paradigm—General principles. *Nature Clinical Practice Oncology, 4,* 86–100. https://doi.org/10.1038/ncponc0714

Shaib, W.L., Nammour, J.P.A., Gill, H., Mody, M., & Saba, N.F. (2016). The future prospects of immune therapy in gastric and esophageal adenocarcinoma. *Journal of Clinical Medicine, 5,* 100. https://doi.org/10.3390/jcm5110100

Shapiro, J., van Lanschot, J.J.B., Hulshof, M., van Hagen, P., van Berge Henegouwen, M.I., Wijnhoven, B.P.L., ... van der Gaast, A. (2015). Neoadjuvant chemoradiotherapy plus surgery versus surgery alone for oesophageal or junctional cancer (CROSS): Long-term results of a randomised controlled trial. *Lancet Oncology, 16,* 1090–1098. https://doi.org/10.1016/S1470-2045(15)00040-6

Shewale, J.B., Correa, A.M., Baker, C.M., Villafane-Ferriol, N., Hofstetter, W.L., Jordan, V.S., ... Swisher, S.G. (2015). Impact of a fast-track esophagectomy protocol on esophageal cancer patient outcomes and hospital charges. *Annals of Surgery, 261,* 1114–1123. https://doi.org/10.1097/SLA.0000000000000971

Siddiqui, U.D., Banerjee, S., Barth, B., Chauhan, S.S., Gottlieb, K.T., Konda, V., ... Rodriguez, S.A. (2013). Tools for endoscopic stricture dilation. *Gastrointestinal Endoscopy, 78,* 391–404. https://doi.org/10.1016/j.gie.2013.04.170

Siewert, J.R., Stein, H.J., & Feith, M. (2006). Adenocarcinoma of the esophago-gastric junction. *Scandinavian Journal of Surgery, 95,* 260–269. https://doi.org/10.1177/145749690609500409

Surveillance, Epidemiology, and End Results Program. (n.d.). Cancer stat facts: Esophageal cancer. Retrieved from http://seer.cancer.gov/statfacts/html/esoph.html

Swisher, S.G., Hofstetter, W., Komaki, R., Correa, A.M., Erasmus, J., Lee, J.H., ... Ajani, J.A. (2010). Improved long-term outcome with chemoradiotherapy strategies in esophageal cancer. *Annals of Thoracic Surgery, 90,* 892–898. https://doi.org/10.1016/j.athoracsur.2010.04.061

Tsottles, N.D., Lang, P., & Choflet, A.B. (2018). Esophageal cancer. In C.H. Yarbro, D. Wujcik, & B.H. Gobel (Eds.), *Cancer nursing: Principles and practice* (8th ed., pp. 1533–1562). Burlington, MA: Jones & Bartlett Learning.

Turati, F., Negri, E., & La Vecchia, C. (2014). Family history and the risk of cancer: Genetic factors influencing multiple cancer sites. *Expert Review of Anticancer Therapy, 14,* 1–4. https://doi.org/10.1586/14737140.2014.863713

van Boeckel, P.G., & Siersema, P.D. (2015). Refractory esophageal strictures: What to do when dilation fails. *Current Treatment Options in Gastroenterology, 13,* 47–58. https://doi.org/10.1007/s11938-014-0043-6

van Hagen, P., Hulshof, M.C., van Lanschot, J.J., Steyerberg, E.W., van Berge Henegouwen, M.I., Wijnhoven, B.P., ... van der Gaast, A. (2012). Preoperative chemoradiotherapy for esophageal or junctional cancer. *New England Journal of Medicine, 366,* 2074–2084. https://doi.org/10.1056/NEJMoa1112088

Verma, V., Lin, S.H., Simone, C.B., 2nd, & Mehta, M.P. (2016). Clinical outcomes and toxicities of proton radiotherapy for gastrointestinal neoplasms: A systematic review. *Journal of Gastrointestinal Oncology, 7,* 644–664. https://doi.org/10.21037/jgo.2016.05.06

Wainwright, D., Donovan, J.L., Kavadas, V., Cramer, H., & Blazeby, J.M. (2007). Remapping the body: Learning to eat again after surgery for esophageal cancer. *Qualitative Health Research, 17,* 759–771. https://doi.org/10.1177/1049732307302021

Wu, A.J., Bosch, W.R., Chang, D.T., Hong, T.S., Jabbour, S.K., Kleinberg, L.R., ... Goodman, K.A. (2015). Expert consensus contouring guidelines for intensity modulated radiation therapy in esophageal and gastroesophageal junction cancer. *International Journal of Radiation Oncology, Biology, Physics, 92,* 911–920. https://doi.org/10.1016/j.ijrobp.2015.03.030

Xu, Y.J., Cheng, J.C., Lee, J.M., Huang, P.M., Huang, G.H., & Chen, C.C. (2015). A walk-and-eat intervention improves outcomes for patients with esophageal cancer undergoing neoadjuvant chemoradiotherapy. *Oncologist, 20,* 1216–1222. https://doi.org/10.1634/theoncologist.2015-0178

Yang, G.Y., McClosky, S.A., & Khushalani, N.I. (2009). Principles of modern radiation techniques for esophageal and gastroesophageal junction cancers. *Gastrointestinal Cancer Research, 3*(Suppl. 2), S6–S10.

Zablotska, L.B., Chak, A., Das, A., & Neugut, A.I. (2005). Increased risk of squamous cell esophageal cancer after adjuvant radiation therapy for primary breast cancer. *American Journal of Epidemiology, 161,* 330–337. https://doi.org/10.1093/aje/kwi050

Zakko, L., Lutzke, L., & Wang, K.K. (2017). Screening and preventive strategies in esophagogastric cancer. *Surgical Oncology Clinics of North America, 26,* 163–178. https://doi.org/10.1016/j.soc.2016.10.004

CHAPTER 3

Gastric Cancer

Cheryl Pfennig, MSN, RN, NP-C, AOCNP®, and Lisa Parks, MS, ANP-BC

Introduction

Despite its worldwide decline in the past century, gastric cancer remains a major source of cancer deaths around the globe. This chapter will discuss the incidence, epidemiology, screening, prevention, and surveillance of gastric cancer. Survival and mortality, signs and symptoms, and treatment and its implications on clinical nursing will be reviewed as well.

Incidence and Epidemiology

Gastric cancer is the fourth most common cancer worldwide and the second most common cause of cancer-related deaths (Liu, Peng, Yang, Huang, & Li, 2018). More than 950,000 new diagnoses and 720,000 deaths occur annually (Van Cutsem, Sagaert, Topal, Haustermans, & Prenen, 2016). Gastric cancers are categorized by site of origin: gastroesophageal junction (GEJ), proximal stomach, and distal stomach (body and antrum). The incidence of GEJ cancer has increased worldwide because of widespread occurrence of gastroesophageal reflux, Barrett's esophagus, and *Helicobacter pylori* infection (Orditura, Galizia, Lieto, De Vita, & Ciardiello, 2015). In the United States, risk factors for the development of gastric cancer include male sex, non-White race, and older age. The overall five-year relative survival rate in people with gastric cancer in the United States is approximately 29% (Amin et al., 2017).

Etiology and Risk Factors

Risk factors associated with gastric cancer are multifactorial and include those that contribute to chronic gastritis, atrophy, and inflammation such as chronic *H. pylori* infection; pernicious anemia; diets high in salt and salt-preserved foods, nitrates, nitrites, fried foods, processed meats, and alcohol; and diets low in vegetables. In fact, diets high in fruits, vegetables, and fiber are protective against gastric cancer (Ang & Fock, 2014). Other factors include obesity, smoking, prior gastric surgery, prior abdominal radiation, male sex, African American race, and inherited germline mutations in *TP53*, *BRCA2*, and *CDH1* (Karimi, Islami, Anandasabapathy, Freedman, & Kamangar, 2014; Peleteiro, Lopes, Figueiredo, & Lunet, 2011).

Controllable risk factors for gastric cancer include dietary choices. Diets high in fried food, red meat, processed meat and fish, and alcohol (and diets low in vegetables, fruits, milk, and vitamin A) have been associated with an increased risk of gastric carcinoma in several epidemiologic studies (Karimi et al., 2014; Zhu et al., 2013). In 2015, the World Health Organization's International Agency for Research on Cancer concluded a positive association exists between consumption of processed meat and stomach cancer (Bouvard et al., 2015). The risk of gastric cancer increases with a high intake of salt and various salt-preserved foods such as salted fish, cured meat, and salted vegetables (Karimi et al., 2014). Consumption of fruits and vegetables, particularly fruit, has been found to protect against gastric cancer, likely related to the vitamin C content, which reduces the formation of carcinogenic N-nitroso compounds inside the stomach (Ang & Fock, 2014; Yoon & Kim, 2015). Cooked vegetables do not show the same protective effect as raw vegetables (Ang & Fock, 2014; Yoon & Kim, 2015).

An additional modifiable risk factor is body mass index. Excess body weight and obesity are linked with an increased risk of gastric cancer. The strength of the association also increases with increasing body mass index (Karimi et al., 2014; Turati, Tramacere, La Vecchia, & Negri, 2013).

Studies have demonstrated a clear association between *H. pylori* infection and gastric adenocarcinoma related to bacterial properties and host response. *H. pylori* can cause chronic active gastritis and atrophic gastritis, which are early steps in the carcinogenesis sequence (Karimi et al., 2014; Marqués-Lespier, González-Pons, & Cruz-Correa, 2016).

Additional risks include prior exposure to radiation therapy. Adult survivors of testicular cancer and Hodgkin lymphoma, as well as childhood cancer survivors who received abdominal radiation therapy, have demonstrated increased incidence of gastric cancer (Henderson et al., 2012).

One nonmodifiable risk factor is sex. Gastric cancer incidence rates are consistently lower in women than men in both high- and low-risk regions worldwide. Data support the hypothesis that reproductive hormones may have a protective role in gastric cancer risk in women (Z. Wang et al., 2016).

Although most gastric cancers are sporadic, hereditary (familial) gastric cancer accounts for 1%–3% of the global burden of gastric cancer and comprises at least three major syndromes: hereditary diffuse gastric cancer (HDGC), gastric adenocarcinoma and proximal polyposis of the stomach, and familial intestinal gastric cancer. The risk of developing gastric cancer is high in families with these syndromes, but only HDGC has a clear genetic link (Oliveira, Pinheiro, Figueiredo, Seruca, & Carneiro, 2015).

Signs and Symptoms

Gastric cancer can go undetected because patients often are asymptomatic; therefore; it typically is discovered incidentally on endoscopy for evaluation of other issues. Gastric cancer can have a varied presentation and often has no outward physical manifestations until the disease has become at least locally advanced (Van Cutsem et al., 2016). Most often, patients present with symptoms that are vague and often overlooked, as they can be attributed to other issues such as gastroesophageal reflux disease. However, reflux associated with gastric cancer often is unrelieved by traditional reflux treatments. Additional clinical signs and symptoms of gastric cancer include unintentional weight loss, tumor-related anorexia, nausea, persistent vague epigastric abdominal pain, early satiety, and dysphagia, which is especially common with proximal tumors.

Another presenting symptom is change in bowel habits. Patients may report melena or black, tarry stools; constipation (especially if treating pain, nausea, or anemia); and change in nature or pattern of bowel habits. Fatigue is commonly seen in patients secondary to anemia from friable tumors, with a syncopal episode being the trigger for evaluation and diagnosis in many otherwise asymptomatic patients (Van Cutsem et al., 2016; L. Wang et al., 2015). Occult gastrointestinal (GI) bleeding with or without iron-deficiency anemia is not uncommon, whereas overt bleeding (i.e., melena or hematemesis) occurs in less than 20% of cases (Van Cutsem et al., 2016; L. Wang et al., 2015).

Weight loss usually results from insufficient caloric intake and can be attributed to anorexia, nausea, abdominal pain, early satiety, or dysphagia. When present, abdominal pain tends to be epigastric, vague, and mild early in the disease but more severe and constant as the disease progresses.

Gastric fullness (early satiety), dyspepsia lasting more than four weeks, and progressive loss of appetite can be presenting symptoms.

Patients often report nausea or early satiety from the tumor mass or, in cases of an aggressive form of diffuse-type gastric cancer called linitis plastica, from poor distensibility of the stomach. They may also present with a gastric outlet obstruction from an advanced distal tumor.

Patients can also present with signs or symptoms of distant metastatic disease. The most common metastatic sites are the liver, peritoneal surfaces, and nonregional or distant lymph nodes. The presence of a palpable abdominal mass is uncommon and generally indicates long-standing, advanced disease (Correa, 2013). Less commonly, ovarian, central nervous system, bone, pulmonary, or soft tissue metastases can occur. Peritoneal spread can present in premenopausal women with an enlarged ovary, known as a Krukenberg tumor (Cho et al., 2015).

Ascites may be the first indication of peritoneal carcinomatosis. A palpable liver mass can indicate metastasis, although metastatic disease to the liver is often multifocal or diffuse. Liver involvement is often, but not always, associated with an elevation in the serum alkaline phosphatase concentration. Jaundice or clinical evidence of liver failure is seen in the end stages of metastatic disease (Maeda, Kobayashi, & Sakamoto, 2015).

Diagnostic Evaluation

Diagnostic evaluation of suspected gastric cancer should include a complete history and physical examination. Focused areas of the physical examination should include unintentional weight loss and heart rate. Tachycardia is suggestive of dehydration secondary to poor oral intake. Pale oral mucosa is suggestive of anemia, and white patches on the tongue are evidence of thrush. Nurses should examine and palpate the neck and cervical nodal chains for adenopathy. The abdominal examination should include evaluation for abdominal distension; assessment of the nature of skin and subcutaneous tissue; auscultation of the abdomen; evaluation of abdominal firmness; evaluation for nodularity in the umbilical area, which can be indicative of a Sister Mary Joseph nodule; and palpation of the abdomen for hepatosplenomegaly (Mealie & Manthey, 2017).

Laboratory tests include complete blood count (CBC), chemistry panel, and liver function tests. Carcinoembryonic antigen (CEA) can be used to detect tumor metastasis and is associated with gastric cancer prognosis. A systematic review of serum markers for gastric cancer found that elevated CEA levels in patients with gastric cancer were associated with poorer prognosis in terms of disease-free survival (Deng et al., 2015).

Gastric cancer is separated anatomically into true gastric adenocarcinomas (noncardia gastric cancers) and GEJ adenocarcinomas (cardia gastric cancers) (Van Cutsem et al., 2016). Esophagogastroduodenoscopy (EGD) is necessary for tissue diagnosis and anatomic localization of the primary tumor. Endoscopic ultrasound (EUS) should be performed to determine tumor stage and nodal status in the absence of radiographic evidence of distant metastatic disease. Diagnostic laparoscopy with biopsy and peritoneal lavage is performed to evaluate for radiographically occult metastatic disease and carcinomatosis.

Histology

Gastric cancers are categorized by site of occurrence: GEJ, proximal stomach, and distal stomach (body and antrum). Approximately 95% of gastric cancers are adenocarcinomas (Correa, 2013). Lymphoma, carcinoid, leiomyosarcoma, GI stromal tumor, and adenosquamous and squamous cell carcinoma comprise the remaining 5% (Correa, 2013). Gastric adenocarcinoma has two main variants. The most frequent is intestinal type, named because of its similarity to adenocarcinomas arising in the intestinal tract. The less common variant is diffuse-type gastric cancers, characterized by a lack of intercellular adhesions. HDGC is a germline mutation in the cell adhesion protein E-cadherin (*CDH1*) gene. This mutation causes a lack of intercellular adhesions and is inherited as an autosomal dominant trait. The cumulative risk of gastric cancer is 70% by age 80 for *CDH1* mutation carriers (van der Post et al., 2015).

Unlike diffuse gastric cancer, the molecular sequence of progression to an intestinal-type adenocarcinoma is not fully understood. The precancerous stages of the intestinal type are the result of a complex process that results in morphologic transformation of normal mucosa caused by atrophy, inflammation, or loss of cellular differentiation (Correa, 2013). One proposed model for the development of intestinal-type gastric cancer describes a progression from chronic gastritis to chronic atrophic gastritis, intestinal metaplasia, dysplasia, and eventually adenocarcinoma (Correa, 2013). Most patients diagnosed with high-grade dysplasia of the gastric mucosa either already have or will soon develop gastric cancer (Karimi et al., 2014).

Clinical Staging

Tumors involving the GEJ with the tumor epicenter no more than 2 cm into the proximal stomach are staged as esophageal cancers. GEJ tumors with their epicenter located more than 2 cm into the proximal stomach are staged as stomach cancers, even if they involve the GEJ (In et al., 2017). The T categories for gastric cancer correspond to the T categories of esophageal and bowel cancers. EUS is the most reliable nonsurgical method available for evaluating the depth of invasion of primary gastric cancers to define T stage, particularly for early (T1) tumors. The eighth edition of the *AJCC Cancer Staging Manual* classifies T1 as tumor that invades the lamina propria, muscularis mucosae, or submucosa. T2 tumor invades the muscularis propria, T3 tumor penetrates the subserosal connective tissue without invasion of the visceral peritoneum or adjacent structures, and T4 tumor invades the visceral peritoneum or adjacent structures (see Figure 3-1). N1 is one to two positive nodes, N2 is three to six positive nodes, and N3 is seven or more positive nodes. Positive peritoneal cytology is classified as M1 disease (Liu et al., 2018).

A major problem in diagnosis is the identification of patients early, when they are potentially curable. In the United States, two-thirds of patients present with stage III or IV disease, whereas only 10% have stage I disease at the time of diagnosis (Lawson, Sicklick, & Fanta, 2011). In about 5% of primary gastric cancers, a broad region of the gastric wall or even the entire stomach is extensively infiltrated by malignancy, resulting in a rigid thickened stomach, termed *linitis plastica* (Jafferbhoy, Shiwani, & Rustum, 2013). Linitis plastica has an extremely poor prognosis, the potential for early spread and advanced stage at diagnosis, and, because of its diffuse nature, the frequent presence of microscopic disease at surgical margins (Jafferbhoy et al., 2013).

Treatment

After tissue diagnosis and staging evaluation, the National Comprehensive Cancer Network® (NCCN®, 2018) guidelines recommend treatment based on clinical stage. If radiographically evident distant metastatic disease exists, treatment is systemic chemotherapy with palliative intent or a clinical trial. Localized early-stage disease, however, may be treated definitively with endoscopic resection with either endoscopic mucosal resection (EMR) or endoscopic submucosal dissection (ESD). Tumor stage T2 (growing into the muscularis propria) and greater without radiographic evidence of distant disease may benefit from upfront systemic therapy. To rule out radiographically occult metastatic disease, staging laparoscopy is performed surgically prior to initiation of systemic therapy.

Staging laparoscopy is more invasive than computed tomography (CT) or EUS but allows surgeons to directly visualize the liver surface, peritoneum, and local lymph nodes, permitting peritoneal cytology as well as biopsy of any suspicious lesions. At laparoscopy, peritoneal metastases are documented in 20%–30% of Western patients with gas-

Chapter 3. Gastric Cancer 77

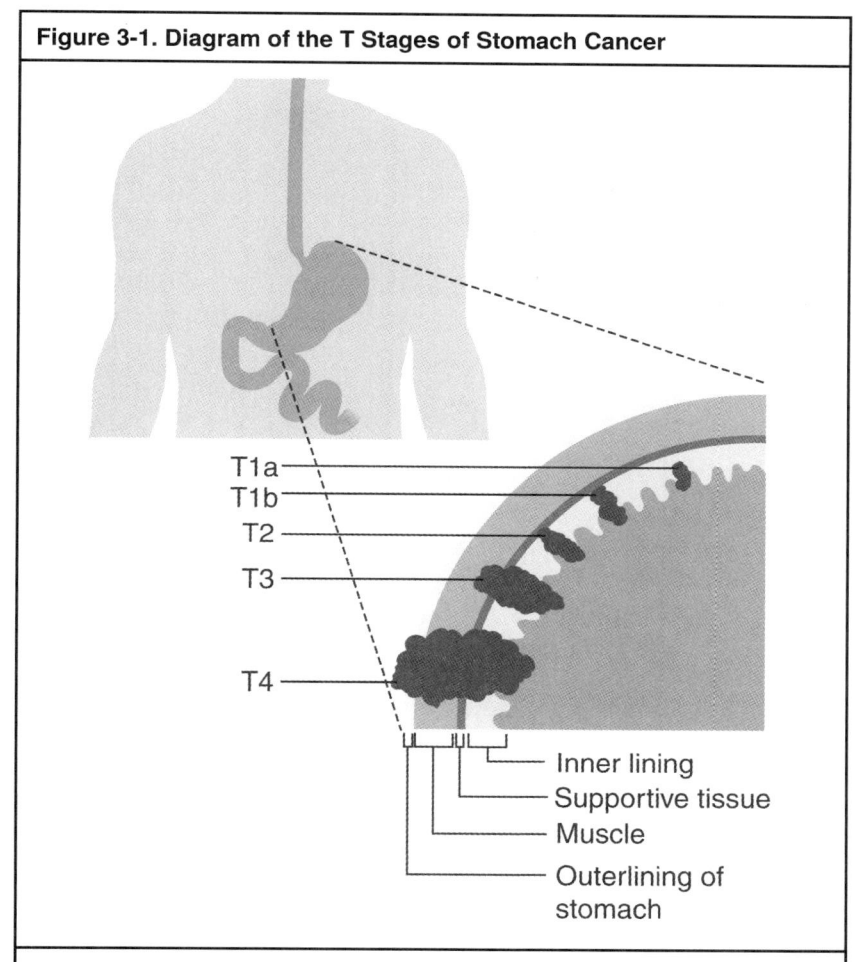

Figure 3-1. Diagram of the T Stages of Stomach Cancer

- Inner lining
- Supportive tissue
- Muscle
- Outerlining of stomach

Note. Image courtesy of Cancer Research UK/Wikimedia Commons. Retrieved from https://commons.wikimedia.org/wiki/File:Diagram_showing_the_T_stages_of_stomach_cancer_CRUK_374.svg. Used under the Creative Commons Attribution-ShareAlike 4.0 International (CC BY-SA 4.0) license (https://creativecommons.org/licenses/by-sa/4.0/legalcode).

tric cancer who have a negative CT (Leake et al., 2012; Simon et al., 2016).

If no evidence of metastatic spread is present, patients will receive neoadjuvant chemotherapy. Chemoradiation in the perioperative period is also considered and includes 5-fluorouracil (5-FU)/capecitabine and concurrent 45 Gy radiation therapy subsequently followed by gastric resection with lymphadenectomy. Following R0 resection, patients will continue with surveillance (NCCN, 2018).

Chemotherapy

Although complete surgical resection can be curative, long-term outcomes are not satisfactory with resection alone, even if microscopically complete (R0). The poor long-term survival rates after surgery alone for patients with gastric and GEJ cancer have led to investigation of adjuvant (postoperative) and neoadjuvant (preoperative) treatment strategies incorporating chemotherapy with or without radiation therapy. Multimodality treatment improves outcomes and has become a standard approach for patients with T2 and higher or node-positive adenocarcinoma of the GEJ. Combined-modality therapy has demonstrated survival benefit over time.

The Adjuvant Chemoradiation Therapy in Stomach Cancer (ARTIST) trial addressed the question of whether adjuvant chemoradiation benefits patients with adequate surgical lymph clearance. Results suggested radiation therapy is beneficial for locoregional control and only patients with node-positive disease benefit from adjuvant chemoradiation (Choi, Kim, & Chao, 2015).

In the largest and most influential gastric cancer treatment trial, the Medical Research Council Adjuvant Gastric Infusional Chemotherapy (MAGIC) trial, 503 patients with potentially resectable gastric (74%), lower esophageal (15%), or GEJ adenocarcinomas (11%) were randomly assigned to surgery alone or surgery plus perioperative chemotherapy consisting of three preoperative and three postoperative cycles of epirubicin, cisplatin, and infusional 5-FU (Choi et al., 2015). In this study, more chemotherapy-treated patients with gastric cancer who underwent radical surgery had a potentially curative procedure (79% vs. 70%) and significantly more had T1 or T2 tumors (52% vs. 37%) and N0 or N1 disease (84% vs. 71%). Challenges with the perioperative chemotherapeutic approach were that only 42% of patients studied were able to complete the treatment protocol, including surgery and all three additional postoperative chemotherapy courses. Reasons cited for incomplete therapy were related to nutritional challenges of receiving chemotherapy following surgical resection. Progression-free survival and overall survival were significantly worse in the surgery-alone group. The 25% reduction in the risk of death favoring chemotherapy translated into an improvement in five-year survival from 23% to 36%. Local failure occurred in 14% of the chemotherapy-treated patients compared with 21% of those undergoing surgery alone, whereas distant metastases developed in 24% and 37% of patients, respectively (Choi et al., 2015).

Preoperative (neoadjuvant) systemic chemotherapy followed by chemoradiation, a treatment break, then surgery has shown pathologic complete response in 20% of patients in a phase 2 clinical trial of patients with localized gastric cancer (Badgwell, Das, & Ajani, 2017). Approximately 85% of patients completed the prescribed course of chemotherapy and chemoradiation preoperatively (Badgwell et al., 2017). Therapy adherence and completion rates make neoadjuvant therapy appealing, with the goals of higher R0 resection rate and better overall survival. A meta-analysis comparing a variety of preoperative chemotherapy regimens versus surgery alone concluded that neoadjuvant chemotherapy was associated with a statistically significant benefit in terms of overall survival (Schuhmacher et al., 2010; Xiong, Cheng, Ma, & Zhang, 2014). Furthermore, neoadjuvant chemotherapy was associated with a significantly higher R0 tumor resection rate and did not significantly worsen rates of operative complications, perioperative mortality, or grade 3 or 4 adverse effects (Schuhmacher et al., 2010; Xiong et al., 2014).

The most effective chemotherapy regimen has not been conclusively established. Practice is variable, and clinical trials looking at varying regimens and timing are ongoing. NCCN guidelines recommend systemic therapy regimens for advanced gastric cancers, chosen based on patients' performance status, comorbidities, and the drug toxicity profile. First-line therapies recommended by NCCN include using a fluoropyrimidine (5-FU or capecitabine) and a platinum (cisplatin or oxaliplatin). Other first-line regimens include combinations of paclitaxel, carboplatin, docetaxel, irinotecan, and epirubicin (NCCN, 2018).

Side effects from chemotherapy are related to the specific agents used and vary by patient. Platinum-based agents are associated with neurotoxicities. Cisplatin specifically can cause peripheral neuropathy, ototoxicity (hearing impairment and tinnitus), Raynaud phenomenon, myelotoxicity, and encephalopathy (Argyriou, Bruna, Marmiroli, & Cavaletti, 2012). Administration of oxaliplatin may lead to an acute neurosensory complex within 24–72 hours after each dose, with patients developing sensitivity to touching cold objects; paresthesias and dysesthesias of the hands, feet, and perioral region; unusual cold-induced pharyngolaryngeal dysesthesias; and muscle cramps. Symptoms generally recur with each dose (Argyriou et al., 2013).

Many patients receiving chemotherapy will describe "chemobrain," or a cognitive delay comprising trouble processing or recalling, a delay in thinking, diminished attention span, or reduced short-term memory. The true mechanism of this is unknown and thought to be multifactorial (Wefel, Kesler, Noll, & Schagen, 2015).

Immunotherapy

The prerequisite for effective antitumor immune-based treatment is the stimulation of a cancer-specific immune response. Three of the most widely studied therapies are the monoclonal antibodies (mAbs) anti–epidermal growth factor receptor (anti-EGFR), anti-HER2, and anti–vascular endothelial growth factor (anti-VEGF). EGFR promotes and modulates via tyrosine kinase apoptosis and proliferation. Existing anti-EGFR treatment for gastric cancer consists of oral tyrosine kinase inhibitors (erlotinib, gefitinib) and mAbs (cetuximab, panitumumab, and matuzumab) (Niccolai, Taddei, Prisco, & Amedei, 2015).

HER2 has been shown to be hyperexpressed in GEJ cancer. This expression has been connected to increased invasion and poor response to neoadjuvant chemotherapy or overall reduced survival (Niccolai et al., 2015). The anti-HER2 mAb treatment used in gastric cancer is trastuzumab. Trastuzumab works by blocking HER2 receptor dimerization, favoring the receptor destruction and promoting cytotoxicity (Niccolai et al., 2015).

VEGF hyperexpression correlates with a poor prognosis and reduced survival. Bevacizumab is used in gastric cancer and is an antiangiogenic factor. It increases chemotherapy drug delivery and decreases interstitial fluid pressures (Niccolai et al., 2015).

Radiation Therapy

Radiation therapy uses energy to kill malignant cells in the area targeted for treatment. External beam radiation therapy is the modality most often used to treat gastric cancer, with five treatments per week over five weeks, often in combination with a radiosensitizing chemotherapy agent (Ajani et al., 2004). Radiation can be used to kill cancer that cannot be visualized or removed at the time of surgery and may prevent or delay recurrence of disease. Radiation also can help palliate symptoms of gastric cancer such as pain, bleeding, and dysphagia.

Side effects of radiation therapy include skin irritation at the radiation site, nausea, vomiting, diarrhea, fatigue, and bone marrow suppression. These side effects are usually short-lived and subside within a few weeks of completing therapy.

The optimal type, dose, combination, and timing of concurrent chemoradiation has not been well established in gastric cancer (Choi et al., 2015). Preoperative combined chemotherapy and radiation therapy is more commonly used for esophageal, GEJ, and gastric cardia cancers than for potentially resectable noncardia gastric adenocarcinomas.

The Dutch CROSS trial randomly assigned 363 patients with potentially resectable esophageal or GEJ cancer to preoperative chemoradiation versus surgery alone. Preoperative treatment consisted of weekly paclitaxel plus carboplatin plus concurrent radiation therapy over five weeks. Preoperative chemoradiation was well tolerated. The R0 resection rate was higher with chemoradiation (92% vs. 65%), and 29% of those treated with chemoradiation had a pathologic complete response. At follow-up of 32 months, overall survival was significantly better with preoperative chemoradiation (Shapiro et al., 2015; Sjoquist et al., 2011).

The multicenter German POET trial, which was limited to patients with GEJ adenocarcinoma, compared neoadjuvant chemoradiation with induction chemotherapy alone. Although findings showed potentially clinically meaningful survival differences that favored chemoradiation, they were not statistically significant. It is unclear also if these results could be applied for patients with distal gastric cancers (Stahl et al., 2009).

Three separate phase 2 studies using different chemoradiation protocols showed pathologic complete response rates of 20%–30%, and 70%–78% of the patients were able to undergo an R0 resection after chemoradiation. No randomized controlled studies have been performed, so it is unknown whether these results are better than could be achieved with surgery alone, neoadjuvant chemotherapy, or surgery followed by adjuvant chemoradiation (Ajani et al., 2004, 2005, 2006; Badgwell et al., 2017; Yao et al., 2003).

Surgery

Complete surgical resection is the only cure for gastric cancer. Resection offers the best chance for long-term survival for patients with localized gastric cancer, particularly when used in combination with adjuvant or perioperative chemotherapy or chemoradiation (Cunningham et al., 2006). NCCN guidelines recommend that palliative gastric resections be reserved for the palliation of obstructing tumors or uncontrollable bleeding. In these cases, a lymph node dissection is not required (NCCN, 2018).

Gastrectomy is the most widely used approach for therapy of invasive gastric cancer, although superficial cancers can sometimes be treated endoscopically. Endoscopic resection with EMR or ESD of early-stage gastric cancer can be considered adequate therapy when the lesion is less than 2 cm in diameter or is well or moderately well differentiated (Van Cutsem et al., 2016). EMR or ESD for gastric cancers that are poorly differentiated and demonstrate evidence of lymphovascular invasion into the deep submucosa and have positive lateral or deep margins or lymph node metastases should be considered incomplete resections, and additional therapy with gastrectomy should be considered (Ahn et al., 2011). Resectable localized tumors not appropriate for EMR that are limited to the lamina propria, muscularis propria, or submucosa should be completely surgically resected with gastric resection with lymph node resection (NCCN, 2018).

Total gastrectomy, which removes the entire stomach, is usually performed for lesions in the proximal (upper third) of the stomach, whereas partial gastrectomy (distal gastrectomy, subtotal gastrectomy) with resection of adjacent lymph nodes is sufficient for lesions in the distal (lower two-thirds) of the stomach. Patients with large midgastric lesions or infiltrative disease (e.g., linitis plastica) may require total gastrectomy. Quality of life after distal gastrectomy, when anatomically possible, is superior to that after a total gastrectomy (Wu et al., 2008).

Patients undergoing total gastrectomy for malignancy should undergo preoperative staging to rule out metastatic disease, including CT of the abdomen and upper endoscopy, which can be used to evaluate the extent of locoregional disease using ultrasound. This also evaluates the anatomy of the esophagus and stomach, which may affect the type of reconstruction. Staging laparoscopy may be indicated for patients with gastric adenocarcinoma (Van Cutsem et al., 2016).

Gastric cancers are considered unresectable in cases of obvious distant metastases; invasion of a major vascular structure, such as the aorta; or disease encasement or occlusion of the hepatic artery or celiac axis/proximal splenic artery. The presence of linitis plastica is a contraindication to potentially curative resection (Jafferbhoy et al., 2013). However, others have reported that long-term survival in selected patients who undergo optimal resection (negative margins guided by intraoperative frozen section analysis and a D2/D3 lymphadenectomy) is comparable to that in optimally resected patients without linitis plastica (Blackham et al., 2016).

The presence of locoregional lymph node metastases that are located geographically distant from the tumor (e.g., celiac nodes with a primary tumor on the greater curvature of the stomach) should not be considered an indicator of unresectability. Involvement of other intra-abdominal nodal groups (i.e., pancreaticoduodenal, retropancreatic, peripancreatic, superior mesenteric, middle colic, paraaortic, and retroperitoneal) is classified as distant metastasis (In et al., 2017). Lymph nodes behind or inferior to the pancreas, in the aortocaval region, into the mediastinum, or in the porta hepatis are typically considered outside of the surgical field and are considered unresectable. Prophylactic splenectomy is not required, but splenectomy may be performed if the spleen or splenic hilum is involved. In splenectomy cases, postsplenectomy vaccines must be given, and patients must be educated on the increased risk of sepsis after loss of the spleen.

For proximal tumors (Siewert type II), total gastrectomy (esophagojejunostomy) with Roux-en-Y anastomosis and D2 lymphadenectomy is performed. For some mid-body and distal tumors, surgery can be either partial gastrectomy (resecting 75%–80% of the distal stomach) with Roux-en-Y reconstruction or loop gastrojejunostomy (Billroth II) with D2 lymphadenectomy. No differences in risks exist based on various therapy approaches (Zollinger & Ellison, 2011).

Thus, total gastrectomy is the preferred surgical resection for proximal gastric tumors (Pu et al., 2013). Tumors of the proximal stomach that do not invade the GEJ can be approached by either a total gastrectomy or a proximal subtotal gastrectomy. Total gastrectomy is the most common surgery performed, largely because the Roux-en-Y reconstruction performed during total gastrectomy has an extremely low incidence of reflux esophagitis (Van Cutsem et al., 2016). In comparison, approximately one-third of patients develop reflux esophagitis after a proximal subtotal gastrectomy (Van Cutsem et al., 2016). Decreased ability to work and overall malaise in patients with proximal gastric resection secondary to reflux symptoms and anastomotic stenosis can affect quality of life (Pu et al., 2013).

Total gastrectomy surgical reconstruction optimally would preserve duodenal function, preventing loss of fat-soluble vitamins and impact on duodenal peristalsis. Pouch reconstruction has better functional outcomes and improved quality of life compared with other types of reconstruction (El Halabi & Lawrence, 2008). Patients who have had a gastric pouch reconstruction have a decreased incidence of dumping syndrome and improved quality of life compared with patients who did not undergo pouch reconstruction (El Halabi & Lawrence, 2008). Pouch reconstruction, regardless of type, did not increase morbidity or mortality, length of operation, or length of hospital stay (El Halabi & Lawrence, 2008). In one study, patients with pouch reconstruction regained preoperative quality of life within two years of their gastrectomy, compared with five years for those without pouch reconstruction (Fein et al., 2008).

Total gastrectomy usually is accomplished via a midline laparotomy by exposing and isolating the stomach, dividing the esophagus and proximal duodenum, removing the specimen, and then restoring GI continuity. For most patients undergoing total gastrectomy, intraoperative frozen sections of the proximal or distal margins are obtained. For adenocarcinoma, the margins should be clear of tumor. For patients undergoing total gastrectomy for gastric adenocarcinoma or carcinoid, D1 lymphadenectomy is performed, rather than a lesser (D0) or greater amount (D2). A more extended lymphadenectomy increases perioperative morbidity and mortality of an already potentially morbid operation. A jejunal feeding tube (J-tube) may be placed approximately 20 cm distal to the Roux-en-Y jejunojejunostomy (Dann et al., 2015). The J-tube provides enteral access for early enteral feeding, as well as delivery of medications in the postoperative period. The routine use of jejunal feeding tubes, however, is controversial, because data are conflicting as to whether it increases or decreases the morbidity of the procedure (Sun et al., 2016).

The primary focus in the postoperative inpatient setting is nutrition, pain control, monitoring of laboratory work, wound care, and early ambulation. Routine blood work including CBC with differential, electrolyte panel, blood urea nitrogen, and creatinine must be monitored for anemia, infection, electrolyte imbalance, and kidney function. The incision site is monitored daily for signs of infection and proper healing. Following gastrectomy, patients will have a nasogastric tube. Once patients show no evidence of anastomotic leak, the nasogastric tube is removed. Supplemental jejunostomy tube feedings will begin on postoperative day 1 and will continue until oral intake is adequate. Oral feeding is started four to seven days postoperatively (Russell, Hsu, & Mansfield, 2012). Upper GI studies are done as indicated (e.g., fever, tachycardia, tachypnea, leukocytosis). Approximately 10% of patients develop dumping syndrome, which consists of diaphoresis, abdominal cramps, and watery diarrhea after intake of highly concentrated sweets and hyperosmolar liquids (Fein et al., 2008). Early ambulation reduces risk of postoperative pneumonia, ileus, and thrombosis. Patients will be in a hypercoagulable state; prophylactic low-molecular-weight heparin is started postoperatively and continued for 28 days (Lyman et al., 2013).

A swallow study can be performed to evaluate the esophagojejunal anastomosis for anastomotic leak prior to initiating an oral diet. In the absence of anastomotic leak, a liquid diet is started and advanced as tolerated. Small, frequent meals that are high in protein and include fat should be consumed approximately six times per day. Liquids may need to be taken separately from solids. Meals high in simple carbohydrates can contribute to dumping syndrome and may need to be avoided.

The initial evaluation for most patients presenting with postoperative GI symptoms is abdominal CT. Immediate postoperative surgical complications following total gastrectomy are primarily the result of consequences of anastomotic leak (Newman & Mulholland, 2006). Disruption of the esophagojejunal anastomosis is the most serious complication in the early postoperative period. Minor leaks without systemic sepsis can be managed conservatively with antibiotics, intestinal decompression, and percutaneous drainage of any associated fluid collections or abscess. Intestinal decompression in the absence of the stomach is accomplished using a nasogastric tube placed into the jejunum distal to the esophageal anastomosis, typically using fluoroscopic guidance (Guo & Duan, 2012). The occurrence of anastomotic leak increases the risk for subsequent anastomotic stricture. Stricture of the esophagojejunostomy anastomosis occurs in approximately 4% of patients (Fukagawa et al., 2010). Patients with anastomotic stricture will usually present with dysphagia. Upper endoscopy can be used to diagnose the stricture, which also can be dilated endoscopically; however, repeated sessions may be needed.

Dietary intake alterations and weight loss are to be anticipated with this procedure. Close involvement with a dietitian familiar with postgastrectomy patients is recommended to help patients adjust to their new dietary regimen and minimize weight loss. Vitamin and mineral supplementation also is required. A 10%–15% decrease in body weight and postgastrectomy syndromes are common sequelae of total gastrectomy. Dumping syndrome and diarrhea are most severe in the initial postoperative period and generally improve within 12 weeks (Bolton & Conway, 2011). Complications should be suspected in patients who complain of severe or persistent GI symptoms such as epigastric pain, nausea, vomiting, early satiety, bloating, diarrhea, or weight loss.

Nursing Care

Nursing considerations at diagnosis include a thorough assessment. Nurses should assess for physical findings related to gastric cancer, such as epigastric discomfort, dyspepsia, anorexia, nausea, sense of fullness, gas pains, unusual tiredness, abdominal pains, constipation, weight loss, vomiting, hematemesis, blood in the stool, dysphagia, jaundice, ascites, and bone pain.

Nurses need to educate patients, families, and caregivers by encouraging behavioral modifications including relaxation, exercise programs, occupational therapy, and occasional pharmacologic interventions, such as use of central nervous system stimulants (Sood, Barton, & Loprinzi, 2006).

Fatigue is a common problem in patients with cancer, both among those undergoing active cancer treatment and in survivors who have completed treatment. The most important factors contributing to cancer-related fatigue are progressive tumor growth, treatment with cytotoxic chemotherapy, radiation therapy, anemia, pain, emotional distress, sleep disturbance, and poor nutrition (Gupta, Lis, & Grutsch, 2007).

Chemotherapy-induced nausea and vomiting is a side effect feared by many patients. Counsel patients on this side effect and the prophylactic use of antiemetics, especially when therapy includes highly emetogenic agents such as cisplatin. Immunosuppression is another risk of chemotherapy. Patients need education on bone marrow suppression and nadir. Caution should be used in public places and around sick people. Attention must be given to basic infection control such as handwashing. Granulocyte–colony-stimulating factors may be used to help protect against infections in patients demonstrating neutropenia.

Postoperative nursing considerations include GI decompression (nasogastric tube), irrigation and patency of the tube, assessment of bowel sounds and passage of gas, complaints of nausea, and the amount and description of gastric fluid output. Assessment for complications such as hemorrhage, obstruction, anastomotic leaks, infection, peritonitis, ileus, thrombosis, and pneumonia in the early postoperative period is critical. Nurses should provide comfort measures and administer analgesics as ordered. They also should encourage deep breathing to prevent pulmonary complications, protect patients' skin, and promote comfort. Nasogastric suction should be maintained to remove fluids and gas in the stomach and prevent painful distension. When nasogastric drainage has decreased and bowel sounds have returned, patients can begin oral fluids and progress slowly.

Patient education includes the importance of adherence to palliative and follow-up care. Nurses must ensure that patients understand all medications, including the dosage, route, action, and adverse effects. Education includes the signs and symptoms of infection and how to care for the incision. Nurses should instruct patients to notify the physician if signs of infection occur. They also should encourage patients to seek psychosocial support through local support groups, clergy, or counseling services. If appropriate, palliative care services should be suggested.

Patient education should cover methods to enhance nutritional intake to maintain ideal body weight. Patients may tolerate several small meals a day better than three meals a day. They should take liquid supplements and vitamins as prescribed. A referral to a registered dietitian should be implemented to assist in dietary and supplement teaching. Nurses should teach family members and friends strategies to prevent malnutrition. Strategies include increasing the intake of fresh fruits and vegetables that are high in vitamin C, maintaining adequate intake of protein, and decreasing intake of salty, starchy, smoked, and nitrite-preserved foods.

Prognosis

Prognosis has improved over the past two decades, with improvements attributable to advances in surgical treatment, postoperative care, and multimodality therapy. In the United States, the five-year overall survival rate is 31% (Surveillance, Epidemiology, and End Results Program, n.d.). The high mortality rate reflects the prevalence of advanced disease at presentation and relatively aggressive biology. Early lesions are usually asymptomatic and infrequently detected outside the realm of a screening program. Early-stage gastric cancer has a 90% five-year survival rate (Strong et al., 2015).

An additional contributing factor to the persistently high mortality rate is the change in the distribution of cancers from the body and antrum to the proximal stomach during the past 20 years

(Marqués-Lespier et al., 2016). Cancers involving the proximal stomach and GEJ have increased steadily at a rate exceeding that of any other cancer except melanoma and lung cancer. Aside from a correlation with increasing obesity, the reasons for this are unclear. Cardia gastric cancer and diffuse-type noncardia gastric cancer have the worst prognosis. Few of these cancers are detected at early stages, resulting in low five-year survival rates (Marqués-Lespier et al., 2016).

Prevention

Patients with extensive atrophic or metaplastic changes in the gastric mucosa are at increased risk for gastric cancer (Correa, 2013). Screening should be limited to individuals found to be at high risk for gastric cancer, including those with a genetic predisposition (e.g., hereditary nonpolyposis colorectal cancer, familial polyposis coli, *CDH1* gene mutation, *H. pylori* infection, diagnosed dysplasia such as Barrett's esophagus). Early evaluation of symptomatic patients may increase the likelihood of finding an early tumor (Lawson et al., 2011).

HDGC is inherited as an autosomal dominant trait with high penetrance with germline truncating mutations of the *CDH1* gene, located on chromosome 16q22.1. Lifetime cumulative risk for advanced diffuse-type gastric cancer in *CDH1* mutation carriers has been updated to 70% for men and 56% for women by the age of 80 years (Karimi et al., 2014). The average age at onset of HDGC is 38 years, although it ranges from 14 to 82 years (Hansford et al., 2015). The presence of a *CDH1* mutation in a family is usually recognized when a case of diffuse gastric cancer occurs in a family member younger than 50 years old or when several cases occur in one family. NCCN (2018) guidelines suggest that although most gastric cancers are sporadic, an estimated 5%–10% have a familial component, and 3%–5% are associated with an inherited cancer predisposition syndrome. Genetic risk assessment is recommended for individuals affected with gastric cancer before the age of 40 years or with one or more first- or second-degree relatives with gastric cancer, early-onset breast cancer, or other genetic hereditary syndromes, such as Lynch syndrome (NCCN, 2018).

Surveillance

NCCN guidelines for surveillance vary based on the stage of cancer at diagnosis. For in situ and stage I tumors, surveillance includes history and physical examination every 3–6 months for 1–2 years, every 6–12 months for 3–5 years, and then annually thereafter (NCCN, 2018). Laboratory studies including CBC, chemistry panel, and nutritional deficiencies, such as B_{12} and iron, should be monitored and treated as clinically indicated. Upper endoscopy is recommended for tumors successfully endoscopically resected and should be performed every six months for one year and then annually for three years. For surgically resected tumors, EGD is recommended as needed for symptoms only. Routine CT should be performed as clinically indicated based on symptoms and concern for recurrence (NCCN, 2018).

For stage II and III (or neoadjuvantly treated stage I–III) tumors, NCCN guidelines recommend the same history and physical examination frequency as for stage I tumors. CBC and chemistry profile should be obtained as clinically indicated. Monitor for nutritional issues, such as deficiency in vitamin B_{12} and D, fat malabsorption, and dumping syndrome with assessments of patients' self-report of bowel habits and dietary tolerances, as well as serum levels of iron, ferritin, folate, calcium, phosphorus, magnesium, thiamine, copper, alpha-tocopherol and retinol-binding protein. For patients who have had a partial or total gastrectomy, EGD is recommended as needed for symptoms only. Routine surveillance endoscopy is not necessary. Endoscopy is appropriate when symptoms warrant investigation. Locoregional recurrence of adenocarcinoma in the setting of total gastrectomy is almost universally fatal, and no evidence supports that early detection of recurrence prolongs life. CT of the chest, abdomen, and pelvis with oral and IV contrast should be performed every six months for the first two years and then annually for up to five years (NCCN, 2018).

Survivorship

The American Cancer Society and the American College of Sports Medicine have developed nutrition and physical activity guidelines for cancer survivors based on the available evidence linking diet, weight, and physical activity to cancer outcomes (Schmitz et al., 2010). Key points of the recommendations include maintaining a healthy weight, engaging in at least 30 minutes of moderate to vigorous physical activity five or more days a week, consuming a healthy diet with at least five servings of fruits and vegetables per day, limiting ingestion of processed foods and red meats, and limiting alcohol to no more than one drink per day for women and two drinks per day for men (Rock et al., 2012).

Summary

Gastric adenocarcinoma remains a significant world health issue. Outcomes for patients remain poor because of diagnosis at advanced stages. However, neoadjuvant therapy and immunotherapy continue to offer promising results. The complexities of the disease biology and post-treatment morbidity offer many opportunities for oncology nursing care to improve patient outcomes and quality of life.

References

Ahn, J.Y., Jung, H.-Y., Choi, K.D., Choi, J.Y., Kim, M.-Y., Lee, J.H., ... Park, Y.S. (2011). Endoscopic and oncologic outcomes after endoscopic resection for early gastric cancer: 1370 cases of absolute and extended indications. *Gastrointestinal Endoscopy, 74*, 485–493. https://doi.org/10.1016/j.gie.2011.04.038

Ajani, J.A., Mansfield, P.F., Crane, C.H., Wu, T.T., Lunagomez, S., Lynch, P.M., ... Pisters, P.W. (2005). Paclitaxel-based chemoradiotherapy in localized gastric carcinoma: Degree of pathologic response and not clinical parameters dictated patient outcome. *Journal of Clinical Oncology, 23*, 1237–1244. https://doi.org/10.1200/JCO.2005.01.305

Ajani, J.A., Mansfield, P.F., Janjan, N., Morris, J., Pisters, P.W., Lynch, P.M., ... Gunderson, L.L. (2004). Multi-institutional trial of preoperative chemoradiotherapy in patients with potentially resectable gastric carcinoma. *Journal of Clinical Oncology, 22*, 2774–2780. https://doi.org/10.1200/JCO.2004.01.015

Ajani, J.A., Winter, K., Okawara, G.S., Donohue, J.H., Pisters, P.W., Crane, C.H., ... Rich, T.A. (2006). Phase II trial of preoperative chemoradiation in patients with localized gastric adenocarcinoma (RTOG 9904): Quality of combined modality therapy and pathologic response. *Journal of Clinical Oncology, 24*, 3953–3958. https://doi.org/10.1200/JCO.2006.06.4840

Amin, M.B., Greene, F.L., Edge, S.B., Compton, C.C., Gershenwald, J.E., Brookland, R.K., ... Winchester, D.P. (2017). The eighth edition AJCC Cancer Staging Manual: Continuing to build a bridge from a population-based to a more "personalized" approach to cancer staging. *CA: A Cancer Journal for Clinicians, 67*, 93–99. https://doi.org/10.3322/caac.21388

Ang, T., & Fock, K. (2014). Clinical epidemiology of gastric cancer. *Singapore Medical Journal, 55*, 621–628. https://doi.org/10.11622/smedj.2014174

Argyriou, A.A., Bruna, J., Marmiroli, P., & Cavaletti, G. (2012). Chemotherapy-induced peripheral neurotoxicity (CIPN): An update. *Critical Reviews in Oncology/Hematology, 82*, 51–77. https://doi.org/10.1016/j.critrevonc.2011.04.012

Argyriou, A.A., Cavaletti, G., Briani, C., Velasco, R., Bruna, J., Campagnolo, M., ... Kalofonos, H.P. (2013). Clinical pattern and associations of oxaliplatin acute neurotoxicity: A prospective study in 170 patients with colorectal cancer. *Cancer, 119*, 438–444. https://doi.org/10.1002/cncr.27732

Badgwell, B., Das, P., & Ajani, J. (2017). Treatment of localized gastric and gastroesophageal adenocarcinoma: The role of accurate staging and preoperative therapy. *Journal of Hematology and Oncology, 10*, 149. https://doi.org/10.1186/s13045-017-0517-9

Blackham, A.U., Swords, D.S., Levine, E.A., Fino, N.F., Squires, M.H., Poultsides, G., ... Votanopoulos, K.I. (2016). Is linitis plastica a contraindication for surgical resection: A multi-institution study of the U.S. Gastric Cancer Collaborative. *Annals of Surgical Oncology, 23*, 1203–1211. https://doi.org/10.1245/s10434-015-4947-8

Bolton, J., & Conway, W. (2011). Postgastrectomy syndromes. *Surgical Clinics of North America, 91,* 1105–1122. https://doi.org/10.1016/j.suc.2011.07.001

Bouvard, V., Loomis, D., Guyton, K.Z., Grosse, Y., Ghissassi, F.E., Benbrahim-Tallaa, L., ... Straif, K. (2015). Carcinogenicity of consumption of red and processed meat. *Lancet Oncology, 16,* 1599–1600. https://doi.org/10.1016/S1470-2045(15)00444-1

Cho, J.H., Lim, J.Y., Choi, A.R., Choi, S.M., Kim, J.W., Choi, S.H., & Cho, J.Y. (2015). Comparison of surgery plus chemotherapy and palliative chemotherapy alone for advanced gastric cancer with Krukenberg tumor. *Cancer Research and Treatment, 47,* 697–705. https://doi.org/10.4143/crt.2013.175

Choi, A.H., Kim, J., & Chao, J. (2015). Perioperative chemotherapy for resectable gastric cancer: MAGIC and beyond. *World Journal of Gastroenterology, 21,* 7343–7348. https://doi.org/10.3748/wjg.v21.i24.7343

Correa, P. (2013). Gastric cancer: Overview. *Gastroenterology Clinics of North America, 42,* 211–217. https://doi.org/10.1016/j.gtc.2013.01.002

Cunningham, D., Allum, W.H., Stenning, S.P., Thompson, J.N., Van de Velde, C.J.H., Nicolson, M., ... Chua, Y.J. (2006). Perioperative chemotherapy versus surgery alone for resectable gastroesophageal cancer. *New England Journal of Medicine, 355,* 11–20. https://doi.org/10.1056/NEJMoa055531

Dann, G., Squires, M., Postlewait, L., Kooby, D., Poultsides, G., Weber, S., ... Maithel, S. (2015). An assessment of feeding jejunostomy tube placement at the time of resection for gastric adenocarcinoma: A seven-institution analysis of 837 patients from the U.S. Gastric Cancer Collaborative. *Journal of Surgical Oncology, 112,* 195–202. https://doi.org/10.1002/jso.23983

Deng, K., Yang, L., Hu, B., Wu, H., Zhu, H., & Tang, C. (2015). The prognostic significance of pretreatment serum CEA levels in gastric cancer: A meta-analysis including 14651 patients. *PLOS ONE, 10,* e124151. https://doi.org/10.1371/journal.pone.0124151

El Halabi, H.M., & Lawrence, W., Jr. (2008). Clinical results of various reconstructions employed after total gastrectomy. *Journal of Surgical Oncology, 97,* 186–192. https://doi.org/10.1002/jso.20928

Fein, M., Fuchs, K.H., Thalheimer, A., Freys, S.M., Heimbucher, J., & Thiede, A. (2008). Long-term benefits of Roux-en-Y pouch reconstruction after total gastrectomy: A randomized trial. *Annals of Surgery, 247,* 759–765. https://doi.org/10.1097/SLA.0b013e318167748c

Fukagawa, T., Gotoda, T., Oda, I., Deguchi, Y., Saka, M., Morita, S., & Katai, H. (2010). Stenosis of esophago-jejuno anastomosis after gastric surgery. *World Journal of Surgery, 34,* 1859–1863. https://doi.org/10.1007/s00268-010-0609-y

Guo, S., & Duan, Z. (2012). Decompression of the small bowel by endoscopic long-tube placement. *World Journal of Gastroenterology, 18,* 1822–1826. https://doi.org/10.3748/wjg.v18.i15.1822

Gupta, D., Lis, C.G., & Grutsch, J.F. (2007). The relationship between cancer-related fatigue and patient satisfaction with quality of life in cancer. *Journal of Pain and Symptom Management, 34,* 40–47. https://doi.org/10.1016/j.jpainsymman.2006.10.012

Hansford, S., Kaurah, P., Li-Chang, H., Woo, M., Senz, J., Pinheiro, H., ... Huntsman, D.G. (2015). Hereditary diffuse gastric cancer syndrome: *CDH1* mutations and beyond. *JAMA Oncology, 1,* 23–32. https://doi.org/10.1001/jamaoncol.2014.168

Henderson, T.O., Oeffinger, K.C., Whitton, J., Leisenring, W., Neglia, J., Meadows, A., ... Nathan, P.C. (2012). Secondary gastrointestinal cancer in childhood cancer survivors: A cohort study. *Annals of Internal Medicine, 156,* 757–766. https://doi.org/10.7326/0003-4819-156-11-201206050-00002

In, H., Solsky, I., Palis, B., Langdon-Embry, M., Ajani, J., & Sano, T. (2017). Validation of the 8th edition of the AJCC TNM staging system for gastric cancer using the

National Cancer Database. *Annals of Surgical Oncology, 24,* 3683–3691. https://doi.org/10.1245/s10434-017-6078-x
Jafferbhoy, S., Shiwani, H., & Rustum, Q. (2013). Managing gastric linitis plastica: Keep the scalpel sheathed. *Sultan Qaboos University Medical Journal, 13,* 451–453. Retrieved from https://www.ncbi.nlm.nih.gov/pmc/articles/PMC3749031
Karimi, P., Islami, F., Anandasabapathy, S., Freedman, N., & Kamangar, F. (2014). Gastric cancer: Descriptive epidemiology, risk factors, screening, and prevention. *Cancer Epidemiology, Biomarkers and Prevention, 12,* 700–713. https://doi.org/10.1158/1055-9965.EPI-13-1057
Lawson, J.D., Sicklick, J.K., & Fanta, P.T. (2011). Gastric cancer. *Current Problems in Cancer, 35,* 97–127. https://doi.org/10.1016/j.currproblcancer.2011.03.001
Leake, P.A., Cardoso, R., Seevaratnam, R., Lourenco, L., Helyer, L., Mahar, A., ... Coburn, N.G. (2012). A systematic review of the accuracy and indications for diagnostic laparoscopy prior to curative-intent resection of gastric cancer. *Gastric Cancer, 15*(Suppl. 1), S38–S47. https://doi.org/10.1007/s10120-011-0047-z
Liu, J.-Y., Peng, C.-W., Yang, X.-J., Huang, C.-Q., & Li, Y. (2018). The prognosis role of AJCC/UICC 8th edition staging system in gastric cancer, a retrospective analysis. *American Journal of Translational Research, 10,* 292–303. Retrieved from https://www.ncbi.nlm.nih.gov/pmc/articles/PMC5801367
Lyman, G.H., Khorana, A.K., Kuderer, N.M., Lee, A.Y., Arcelus, J.I., Balaban, E.P., ... Falanga, A. (2013). Venous thromboembolism prophylaxis and treatment in patients with cancer: American Society of Clinical Oncology clinical practice guideline update. *Journal of Clinical Oncology, 31,* 2189–2204. https://doi.org/10.1200/JCO.2013.49.1118
Maeda, H., Kobayashi, M., & Sakamoto, J. (2015). Evaluation and treatment of malignant ascites secondary to gastric cancer. *World Journal of Gastroenterology, 21,* 10936–10947. https://doi.org/10.3748/wjg.v21.i39.10936
Marqués-Lespier, J.M., González-Pons, M., & Cruz-Correa, M. (2016). Current perspectives on gastric cancer. *Gastroenterology Clinics of North America, 45,* 413–428. https://doi.org/10.1016/j.gtc.2016.04.002
Mealie, C.A., & Manthey, D.E. (2017, October 15). Abdominal, exam. In B. Abai, A. Abu-Ghosh, A.B. Acharya, R. Adigun, T.C. Aeby, M. Agarwal, ... E.K. Zinn (Eds.), *StatPearls* [Online book]. Retrieved from https://www.ncbi.nlm.nih.gov/books/NBK459220
National Comprehensive Cancer Network. (2018). *NCCN Clinical Practice Guidelines in Oncology (NCCN Guidelines®): Gastric cancer* [v.2.2018]. Retrieved from https://www.nccn.org/professionals/physician_gls/pdf/gastric.pdf
Newman, E., & Mulholland, M.W. (2006). Prophylactic gastrectomy for hereditary diffuse gastric cancer syndrome. *Journal of the American College of Surgeons, 202,* 612–617. https://doi.org/10.1016/j.jamcollsurg.2005.12.017
Niccolai, E., Taddei, A., Prisco, D., & Amedei, A. (2015). Gastric cancer and the epoch of immunotherapy approaches. *World Journal of Gastroenterology, 21,* 5778–5793. https://doi.org/10.3748/wjg.v21.i19.5778
Oliveira, C., Pinheiro, H., Figueiredo, J., Seruca, R., & Carneiro, F. (2015). Familial gastric cancer: Genetic susceptibility, pathology, and implications for management. *Lancet Oncology, 16,* e60–e70. https://doi.org/10.1016/S1470-2045(14)71016-2
Orditura, M., Galizia, G., Lieto, E., De Vita, F., & Ciardiello, F. (2015). Treatment of esophagogastric junction carcinoma: An unsolved debate. *World Journal of Gastroenterology, 21,* 4427–4431. https://doi.org/10.3748/wjg.v21.i15.4427
Peleteiro, B., Lopes, C., Figueiredo, C., & Lunet, N. (2011). Salt intake and gastric cancer risk according to *Helicobacter pylori* infection, smoking, tumour site and histological type. *British Journal of Cancer, 104,* 198–207. https://doi.org/10.1038/sj.bjc.6605993

Pu, Y.W., Gong, W., Wu, Y.Y., Chen, Q., He, T.F., & Xing, C.G. (2013). Proximal gastrectomy versus total gastrectomy for proximal gastric carcinoma. A meta-analysis on postoperative complications, 5-year survival, and recurrence rate. *Saudi Medical Journal, 34,* 1223–1228.

Rock, C.L., Doyle, C., Demark-Wahnefried, W., Meyerhardt, J., Courneya, K.S., Schwartz, A.L., ... Gansler, T. (2012). Nutrition and physical activity guidelines for cancer survivors. *CA: A Cancer Journal for Clinicians, 62,* 243–274. https://doi.org/10.3322/caac.21142

Russell, M., Hsu, C., & Mansfield, P. (2012). Primary gastric malignancies. In B. Feig (Ed.), *MD Anderson surgical oncology handbook* (5th ed., pp. 270–322). Houston, TX: Wolters Kluwer.

Schmitz, K.H., Courneya, K.S., Matthews, C., Demark-Wahnefried, W., Galvao, D.A., Pinto, B.M., ... Schwartz, A.L. (2010). American College of Sports Medicine roundtable on exercise guidelines for cancer survivors. *Medicine and Science in Sports and Exercise, 42,* 1409–1426. https://doi.org/10.1249/MSS.0b013e3181e0c112

Schuhmacher, C., Gretschel, S., Lordick, F., Reichardt, P., Hohenberger, W., Eisenberger, C.F., ... Schlag, P.M. (2010). Neoadjuvant chemotherapy compared with surgery alone for locally advanced cancer of the stomach and cardia: European Organisation for Research and Treatment of Cancer randomized trial 40954. *Journal of Clinical Oncology, 28,* 5210–5218. https://doi.org/10.1200/JCO.2009.26.6114

Shapiro, J., van Lanschot, J.J.B., Hulshof, M., van Hagen, P., van Berge Henegouwen, M.I., Wijnhoven, B.P.L., ... van der Gaast, A. (2015). Neoadjuvant chemoradiotherapy plus surgery versus surgery alone for oesophageal or junctional cancer (CROSS): Long-term results of a randomised controlled trial. *Lancet Oncology, 16,* 1090–1098. https://doi.org/10.1016/S1470-2045(15)00040-6

Simon, M., Mal, F., Perniceni, T., Ferraz, J.-M., Strauss, C., Levard, H., ... Gayet, B. (2016). Accuracy of staging laparoscopy in detecting peritoneal dissemination in patients with gastroesophageal adenocarcinoma. *Diseases of the Esophagus, 29,* 236–240. https://doi.org/10.1111/dote.12332

Sjoquist, K.M., Burmeister, B.H., Smithers, B.M., Zalcberg, J.R., Simes, R.J., Barbour, A., & Gebski, V. (2011). Survival after neoadjuvant chemotherapy or chemoradiotherapy for resectable oesophageal carcinoma: An updated meta-analysis. *Lancet Oncology, 12,* 681–692. https://doi.org/10.1016/S1470-2045(11)70142-5

Sood, A., Barton, D.L., & Loprinzi, C.L. (2006). Use of methylphenidate in patients with cancer. *American Journal of Hospice and Palliative Care, 23,* 35–40. https://doi.org/10.1177/104990910602300106

Stahl, M., Walz, M.K., Stuschke, M., Lehmann, N., Meyer, H.J., Riera-Knorrenschild, J., ... Wilke, H. (2009). Phase III comparison of preoperative chemotherapy compared with chemoradiotherapy in patients with locally advanced adenocarcinoma of the esophagogastric junction. *Journal of Clinical Oncology, 27,* 851–856. https://doi.org/10.1200/JCO.2008.17.0506

Strong, V., Wu, A., Selby, L., Gonen, M., Hsu, M., Song, K., ... Brennan, M. (2015). Differences in gastric cancer survival between the US and China. *Journal of Surgical Oncology, 112,* 31–37. https://doi.org/10.1002/jso.23940

Sun, Z., Shenoi, M.M., Nussbaum, D.P., Keenan, J.E., Gulack, B.C., Tyler, D.S., ... Blazer, D.G., III. (2016). Feeding jejunostomy tube placement during resection of gastric cancers. *Journal of Surgical Research, 200,* 189–194. https://doi.org/10.1016/j.jss.2015.07.014

Surveillance, Epidemiology, and End Results Program. (n.d.). Cancer stat facts: Stomach cancer. Retrieved from https://seer.cancer.gov/statfacts/html/stomach.html

Turati, F., Tramacere, I., La Vecchia, C., & Negri, E. (2013). A meta-analysis of body mass index and esophageal and gastric cardia adenocarcinoma. *Annals of Oncology, 24,* 609–617. https://doi.org/10.1093/annonc/mds244

Van Cutsem, E., Sagaert, X., Topal, B., Haustermans, K., & Prenen, H. (2016). Gastric cancer. *Lancet, 388,* 2654–2664. https://doi.org/10.1016/S0140-6736(16)30354-3

van der Post, R.S., Vogelaar, I.P., Carneiro, F., Guilford, P., Huntsman, D., Hoogerbrugge, N., ... Fitzgerald, R.C. (2015). Hereditary diffuse gastric cancer: Updated clinical guidelines with an emphasis on germline *CDH1* mutation carriers. *Journal of Medical Genetics, 52,* 361–374. https://doi.org/10.1136/jmedgenet-2015-103094

Wang, L., Wang, X.-A., Hao, J.-Q., Zhang, L.-N., Li, M.-L., Wu, X.-S., ... Dong, P. (2015). Long-term outcomes after radical gastrectomy in gastric cancer patients with overt bleeding. *World Journal of Gastroenterology, 21,* 13316–13324. https://doi.org/10.3748/wjg.v21.i47.13316

Wang, Z., Butler, L.M., Wu, A.H., Koh, W.-P., Jin, A., Wang, R., & Yuan, J.-M. (2016). Reproductive factors, hormone use and gastric cancer risk: The Singapore Chinese Health study. *International Journal of Cancer, 138,* 2837–2845. https://doi.org/10.1002/ijc.30024

Wefel, J.S., Kesler, S.R., Noll, K.R., & Schagen, S.B. (2015). Clinical characteristics, pathophysiology, and management of noncentral nervous system cancer-related cognitive impairment in adults. *CA: A Cancer Journal for Clinicians, 65,* 123–138. https://doi.org/10.3322/caac.21258

Wu, C.-W., Chiou, J.-M., Ko, F.-S., Lo, S.-S., Chen, J.-H., Lui, W.-Y., & Whang-Peng, J. (2008). Quality of life after curative gastrectomy for gastric cancer in a randomised controlled trial. *British Journal of Cancer, 98,* 54–59. https://doi.org/10.1038/sj.bjc.6604097

Xiong, B.-H., Cheng, Y., Ma, L., & Zhang, C.-Q. (2014). An updated meta-analysis of randomized controlled trial assessing the effect of neoadjuvant chemotherapy in advanced gastric cancer. *Cancer Investigation, 32,* 272–284. https://doi.org/10.3109/07357907.2014.911877

Yao, J.C., Mansfield, P.F., Pisters, P.W., Feig, B.W., Janjan, N.A., Crane, C., & Ajani, J.A. (2003). Combined-modality therapy for gastric cancer. *Seminars in Surgical Oncology, 21,* 223–227. https://doi.org/10.1002/ssu.10040

Yoon, H., & Kim, N. (2015). Diagnosis and management of high risk group for gastric cancer. *Gut and Liver, 9,* 5–17. https://doi.org/10.5009/gnl14118

Zhu, H., Yang, X., Zhang, C., Zhu, C., Tao, G., Zhao, L., ... Sun, X. (2013). Red and processed meat intake is associated with higher gastric cancer risk: A meta-analysis of epidemiological observational studies. *PLOS ONE, 8,* e70955. https://doi.org/10.1371/journal.pone.0070955

Zollinger, R.M., & Ellison, E.C. (2011). *Zollinger's atlas of surgical operations* (9th ed.). New York, NY: McGraw-Hill.

CHAPTER 4

Pancreatic Cancer

Jessica MacIntyre, ARNP, NP-C, AOCNP®

Introduction

Pancreatic cancer and intraductal papillary mucinous neoplasms (IPMNs), also called exocrine cancer, are diseases in which malignant (cancer) cells are found in the tissues of the pancreas (National Cancer Institute [NCI], n.d.). The pancreas is located behind the stomach in the upper left abdomen. It is surrounded by other organs, including the small intestine, liver, and spleen. The pancreas has exocrine and endocrine functions. The exocrine function of the pancreas is responsible for digestion, and the endocrine function regulates blood sugar. Endocrine cancers of the pancreas are termed *neuroendocrine tumors* and are reviewed in Chapter 5.

Incidence and Epidemiology

According to the American Cancer Society (ACS, 2018), an estimated 55,440 cases of pancreatic cancer will be diagnosed in the United States in 2018. The highest incidence rates are found in North America (7.4 per 100,000) and Europe (6.8 per 100,000) (International Agency for Research on Cancer, n.d.). Unfortunately, the number of deaths (44,330) almost equals the number of new cases because of the lack of screening and early prevention. It is the 4th leading cause of cancer death in both men and women (ACS, 2018) and the 12th most common cancer in the world, with a global incidence of 2.4–8.6 cases per 100,000 people per year (Ferlay et al., 2015).

Etiology and Risk Factors

Etiology
Despite the high mortality rate associated with pancreatic cancer, its etiology is poorly understood. However, more than 90% of pancreatic

ductal adenocarcinomas (PDACs) are driven by early activating *KRAS* mutations (Lowery et al., 2017). Genetic and environmental risk factors have also been implicated in the development of PDAC (Simoes, Olson, Saldia, & Kurtz, 2017).

Risk Factors

A strong, consistent association exists between tobacco smoking and development of PDAC (Simoes et al., 2017). The risk of pancreatic cancer in cigarette smokers is twice the risk for those who have never smoked (ACS, 2018). Use of smokeless tobacco also increases the risk of developing pancreatic cancer (ACS, 2018). Other risk factors include history of chronic pancreatitis, diabetes mellitus, obesity, and family history of pancreatic cancer.

It remains unclear whether diabetes plays a causative role in the development of pancreatic cancer, whether it is an early manifestation of pancreatic cancer, or whether an underlying genetic or metabolic association affects the development of these conditions (Simoes et al., 2017). When providing a history in clinical practice, patients will occasionally report a new diagnosis of diabetes that preceded the diagnosis of pancreatic cancer. Research is ongoing in this area.

Obesity has been linked to various cancers, but in reference to pancreatic cancer, increased body mass index, and higher abdominal obesity in particular, leads to additional risk of PDAC. Reduction in the prevalence of overweight and obesity is the goal for prevention of pancreatic cancer, as well as other diseases (Simoes et al., 2017).

Pancreatic cancer related to family history typically is seen in 5%–10% of individuals with one affected first-degree relative (Hruban, Canto, Goggins, Schulick, & Klein, 2010). Some germline mutations are associated with higher risk of developing pancreatic cancer. The germline mutation most associated with higher risk is *BRCA2*, which is also associated with higher sensitivity to DNA-damaging agents, such as mitomycin C and cisplatin (Krantz, Yu, & O'Reilly, 2017). Studies in cancer family registries indicate that carriers of *BRCA2* mutations have about two to three times the risk of PDAC, and those with *BRCA1* mutations have approximately 1.6–2.3 times the risk (Simoes et al., 2017). Mutations in *CDKN2A* and *PALB2* also can be seen with familial risk of pancreatic cancer.

Other genetic syndromes associated with pancreatic cancer are familial atypical multiple mole melanoma, Lynch syndrome, hereditary pancreatitis, familial adenomatous polyposis, and Peutz-Jeghers syndrome (Simoes et al., 2017). A thorough family history is important information to collect on initial diagnosis and presentation. Time taken to discuss family history can help screen for potential at-risk family members, which can prevent future cases of pancreatic cancer. Referral to a genetic specialist or counselor may be warranted if the association is strongly related to family history.

Signs and Symptoms

Signs and symptoms of pancreatic cancer can be related to the location of the disease. The pancreas is divided into three main parts: head, body (neck), and tail. Tumors located in the head and body can produce obstructive symptoms such as pruritus, related to obstructive jaundice (mostly noted in skin and sclera). This results in light-colored stools and dark urine due to the lack of bilirubin. Tumors in the head of the pancreas tend to be detected earlier in the course of the disease because of obvious signs of jaundice. Patients with tumors in the tail of the pancreas will present with left upper quadrant or back pain. These symptoms tend to present later in the course of the disease.

The pancreas is located near a set of nerves called the *celiac plexus*, and back pain can be referred from this area (Seicean, 2014). The celiac plexus is a bundle of nerves that surrounds the aorta, the main artery in the abdomen. The pancreas sits in front of this area. A celiac plexus block may be required to palliate pain. This procedure can be performed endoscopically by a gastroenterologist or can be computed tomography (CT) or x-ray guided by an interventional radiologist. The provider uses imaging guidance to insert a needle and inject an anesthetic into the celiac plexus. The procedure has been effective in some patients; however, additional opioids may be required as an adjunct. Pain alleviation has been reported as high as 90% two weeks after and 70%–90% three months after the procedure (Seicean, 2014).

Malabsorption or pancreatic exocrine insufficiency is also a common symptom on initial presentation. Because the tumor diminishes the exocrine function of the pancreas, the ability to digest carbohydrates, fats, and proteins also becomes compromised. This in turn causes excess gas in the form of flatulence; eructation; and floating, greasy stools. Many patients will require prescribed pancreatic enzymes to palliate these symptoms. Patients with a clinical suspicion of pancreatic exocrine insufficiency despite appropriate replacement may need a more thorough nutritional evaluation (National Comprehensive Cancer Network® [NCCN®], 2017).

Some patients will also present with pyloric or gastric outlet obstruction (GOO). Pancreatic cancer is the most common malignancy associated with GOO. About 10%–25% of patients will develop GOO or duodenal obstruction during the course of the disease (Larssen, Medhus, & Hauge, 2009). Symptoms associated with GOO include intractable nausea and vomiting requiring palliation with a duodenal stent via endoscopy. If a duodenal stent cannot be placed, a percutaneous endoscopic gastrostomy tube is an alternative approach. Additionally, for patients undergoing surgery who are deemed to be inoperable, a prophylactic gastrojejunostomy typically is performed to prevent GOO. Two randomized controlled studies found that approximately 20% of patients who did not undergo a prophylactic gastrojejunostomy developed late GOO that required intervention (NCCN, 2017). Acute abdominal distension is another symptom associated with GOO that is visible on examination and worsens with food intake. Patients with GOO commonly attribute their symptoms to their chemotherapy treatment. As a result, symptoms tend to be overlooked. If GOO is left untreated, hospitalization due to dehydration and cachexia may be required.

Diagnostic Evaluation

When suspicion of pancreatic cancer and signs of obstructive jaundice exist, a complete abdominal ultrasound or a CT scan of the abdomen and pelvis is performed. However, with a suspicion of pancreatic cancer, staging imaging should be done during the initial workup to avoid additional and unnecessary imaging examinations. A chest CT may be performed to rule out metastatic disease. CT and magnetic resonance imaging (MRI) appear to have approximately equivalent accuracy in assessing local involvement of a pancreatic lesion, although MRI may be better at determining metastasis, and CT has the advantages of lower cost and greater availability (Toft et al., 2017). If a CT scan is performed, it is recommended to be ordered as a pancreatic protocol with oral and IV contrast when possible. The pancreatic protocol involves taking thinner slices of the pancreas for better visualization. This type of CT scan was shown to change the staging and management of patients with pancreatic adenocarcinoma in 56% of cases retrospectively at one institution (Walters et al., 2011). Additional staging workup can include endoscopic ultrasound (EUS), endoscopic retrograde cholangiopancreatography, liver function tests, and chest imaging (NCCN, 2017). EUS is helpful in the detection of small lesions and for tissue sampling. EUS-guided fine needle aspiration (EUS-FNA) is preferable to CT-guided FNA in patients with resectable disease because of better diagnostic yield and safety, as well as potentially lower risk of peritoneal seeding, compared to the percutaneous approach (NCCN, 2017). Tissue sampling is needed only if the patient has locally advanced disease and is being recommended to start neoadjuvant or palliative treatment. However, it is likely that an initial biopsy may not yield a positive malignant diagnosis. Often, providers receive a diagnosis of atypical cells as the initial pathology result, which is not sufficient to treat a patient. NCCN recommends that at least one repeat biopsy be performed; EUS-FNA with or without a core biopsy at a center with interprofessional expertise is preferred. Other methods can be considered to obtain tissue diagnosis, including intraductal biopsies and percutaneous or laparoscopic approaches. Additionally, a differential diagnosis may need to be ruled out if the diagnosis is not able to be obtained.

The role of positron-emission tomography (PET) scans in the workup of pancreatic cancer is still being investigated. Most insurers will not cover the cost of a PET scan unless it is being used to assess or confirm metastatic disease. With certain scenarios, if patients are allergic to IV iodine or unable to undergo MRI, insurers may approve a PET scan as an alternative imaging modality.

If surgical resection is being considered, a diagnostic laparoscopy may be performed to ensure the absence of peritoneal, capsular, or serosal implants or studding of metastatic tumor on the liver that may have not been identified on a CT scan. Unfortunately, more than 50% of patients present with advanced-stage pancreatic cancer (Lau & Cheung, 2017). Common sites of metastatic disease include the liver, lung, and peritoneum. NCCN (2017) recommends that staging laparoscopy be considered for patients with resectable pancreatic cancer who are considered to be at increased risk for disseminated disease and for patients with borderline resectable disease prior to administration of neoadjuvant therapy.

Other laboratory work to be considered to complete workup includes biomarkers. The biomarker related to pancreatic cancer is CA 19-9, a sialylated Lewis A blood group antigen. Unfortunately, some patients do not express an elevated CA 19-9 biomarker. This is the result of patients having negative undetectable Lewis antigen. As a result, this biomarker should not be relied upon to diagnose pancreatic cancer. CA 19-9 is also expressed in other malignancies and benign medical conditions, such as pancreatitis. The biomarker is useful, however, in showing treatment response prior to imaging, in surveillance, and to decide on change in treatment if an unexpected rise occurs. The biomarker carcinoembryonic antigen also can be tested if CA 19-9 levels are undetectable.

Histology

Pancreatic cancer is divided into malignant and borderline malignant histology. Ductal cell carcinoma comprises 90% of the pancreatic cancer cases (NCI, 2018). The other histologies in the malignant group are treated differently than PDAC and include the following (NCI, 2018):
- Acinar cell carcinoma

- Adenosquamous carcinoma
- Cystadenocarcinoma (serous and mucinous types)
- Giant cell carcinoma
- Invasive adenocarcinoma associated with cystic mucinous neoplasm or IPMN
- Mixed type (ductal-endocrine or acinar-endocrine)
- Mucinous carcinoma
- Pancreatoblastoma
- Papillary cystic neoplasm
- Signet ring cell carcinoma
- Small cell carcinoma (may be a neuroendocrine tumor)
- Unclassified
- Undifferentiated carcinoma

IPMNs are considered premalignant pancreatic lesions characterized by the papillary growth of the ductal epithelium with rich mucin production, which is responsible for cystic segmental or diffuse dilation of the main pancreatic duct or its branches (Pagliari et al., 2017). IPMNs account for 1%–2% of all pancreatic pathologies and frequently affect the head of the pancreas (50%), but also the tail (7%) and uncinate process (4%) (Pagliari et al., 2017). The increase in frequency of IPMNs may reflect the combined effects of radiologic examinations and progress in the recognition of pathology (Pagliari et al., 2017). As a result, these neoplasms are found incidentally on imaging examinations, and patients tend to be asymptomatic. When symptoms are present, they tend to mimic those of chronic pancreatitis (Aşkan, Bağci, Memiş, & Baştürk, 2017). The management of IPMNs is different than management of PDACs in that surgery is recommended, and only surveillance is recommended in the adjuvant setting. Debate exists as to the best approach to monitoring these patients. Many providers will base surveillance on pathologic features. The most important determinant of outcome in the management of patients with IPMNs is whether an associated invasive carcinoma is present (Aşkan et al., 2017). The recurrence rate is also higher (28%–60%) for IPMNs with an invasive component (Aşkan et al., 2017).

Clinical Staging

Staging according to the American Joint Committee on Cancer tumor-node-metastasis staging system is as follows (Kakar, Pawlik, Allen, & Vauthey, 2017):
- Stage 0: Tis N0 M0
- Stage IA: T1 N0 M0
- Stage IB: T2 N0 M0
- Stage IIA: T3 N0 M0
- Stage IIB: T1–T3 N1 M0

- Stage III: T1–3 N2 M0; T4, Any N, M0 (considered unresectable or locally advanced)
- Stage IV: Any T, Any N, M1 (metastatic)

Figure 4-1 shows stage T2 cancer of the pancreas.

Treatment

Surgery

Surgical resection is the mainstay of curative treatment; however, only 15%–20% of patients diagnosed with pancreatic cancer are eligible for upfront surgery (Conroy et al., 2016). Following diagnostic workup, if patients are deemed to be surgical candidates, they are referred to a surgeon. Patients with stage I or II pancreatic cancer are candidates for surgery. It is preferable that patients seek surgical care at a center that

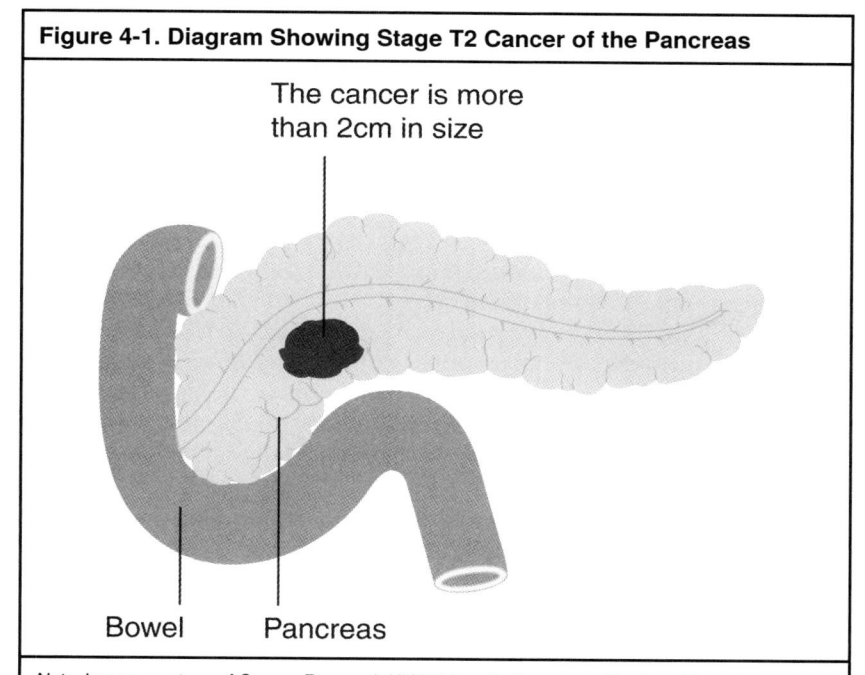

Figure 4-1. Diagram Showing Stage T2 Cancer of the Pancreas

Note. Image courtesy of Cancer Research UK/Wikimedia Commons. Retrieved from https://commons.wikimedia.org/wiki/File:Diagram_showing_stage_T2_cancer_of_the_pancreas_CRUK_254.svg. Used under the Creative Commons Attribution-ShareAlike 4.0 International (CC BY-SA 4.0) license (https://creativecommons.org/licenses/by-sa/4.0/legalcode).

has an interprofessional approach and experience in pancreatic surgeries. NCCN (2017) recommends that pancreatic resections be completed at institutions that perform a large number (at least 15–20 surgeries) of these resections annually.

Depending on the location of the pancreatic cancer, the surgeon will determine what type of surgery to perform. Patients with tumors in the head or neck of the pancreas tend to undergo an open, laparoscopic, or robotic pancreaticoduodenectomy (Whipple) procedure, whereas patients with pancreatic tail tumors will undergo a distal pancreatectomy with splenectomy. If the cancer diffusely involves the pancreas or is present in multiple sites within the pancreas, a total pancreatectomy may be required. Postsurgical pathologic specimen characteristics such as negative margin status (R0 resection), tumor DNA content, tumor size, and absence of lymph node metastasis are the strongest prognostic indicators for long-term patient survival (NCCN, 2017).

Preoperative Management

During the preoperative period, patients may be recommended to undergo additional workup to ensure readiness for surgery. As mentioned previously, a diagnostic laparoscopy may be performed to ensure absence of metastatic disease prior to undergoing surgery. Additional laboratory work, anesthesia clearance (including cardiology and respiratory examinations), and evaluation for bridging coagulation problems should be addressed. Preoperative biliary drainage may be recommended to palliate pruritus and to potentially reduce morbidity by improving liver function preoperatively (NCCN, 2017). Patients should be educated on the typical length of hospital stay and possible postoperative complications. The possibility also exists that the surgery could be aborted intraoperatively if the tumor is found to be unresectable, involving blood vessels or metastatic to other regions. Providing awareness of this to patients will help them understand that surgery may not be definitive, despite the results of the staging workup.

If patients are deemed to be unresectable (unable to have surgery because of vessel involvement) or borderline resectable (interface between the tumor and superior mesenteric artery that is less than 180° of vessel wall involvement), neoadjuvant treatment with chemotherapy or chemoradiation may be recommended to downsize the tumor away from the blood vessels prior to surgical resection to achieve an R0 resection (Conroy et al., 2016).

This may be a time of anxiety for patients because of the period of waiting after the first visit until the time of the surgery. During this time, an interprofessional team will evaluate and reevaluate the case to determine the timing of surgery. Reassuring patients and continuously communicating that precautions are being taken to ultimately improve their safety and outcomes during surgery will provide some relief to patients and caregivers.

Postoperative Management

Variable postoperative complications can develop after pancreatic surgery. Thromboembolic disease risk is high in patients with pancreatic cancer because of its ability to induce the production of inflammatory cytokines that indirectly contribute to the development of hypercoagulability and risk of thromboembolism (Ansari, Ansari, Andersson, & Andrén-Sandberg, 2015). Prophylactic low-molecular-weight heparin should be ordered postsurgery, depending on the patient's history, to prevent a postsurgical embolism. Other postoperative complications include pancreatic leak, fistula formation, pain, and nutrition-related complications. Patients frequently have a jejunostomy tube placed for nutritional support and a nasogastric tube to allow for stomach decompression. Patients with delayed gastric emptying may have total parenteral nutrition including lipids to support them during the initial days to weeks postoperatively. Continuous and accurate nursing assessments of intake and output will allow the surgical team to make critical decisions that will lead patients to a safe recovery. Glucose monitoring is also an important aspect of postsurgical care because a portion of the pancreas has been removed. Assessing glucose levels daily and up to three times a day will allow the medical team to determine if patients require an oral hypoglycemic or insulin prior to discharge.

Communication regarding discharge care is also critical. Depending on the intraoperative findings and preliminary pathology, coordination of postsurgical care at home will be critical for patients to be able to continue their recovery and to be treated with other modalities such as chemotherapy or chemoradiation. It is important to ensure that a follow-up appointment has been secured, as well as a medical oncology appointment.

Chemotherapy

Advances in the treatment of pancreatic cancer have occurred in small increments, bringing modest improvements in survival. No definite standard has been established in the adjuvant treatment of pancreatic cancer. Recently, the ESPAC-4 (European Study Group for Pancreatic Cancer Trial 4) phase 3 randomized trial, which compared gemcitabine combined with capecitabine to gemcitabine alone, indicated that median survival increased from 25.5 months to 28 months (Neoptolemos et al., 2017). Other options that can be considered in the adjuvant setting include 5-fluorouracil (5-FU)/leucovorin, continuous 5-FU, and capecitabine. Additionally, gemcitabine, 5-FU/leucovorin, or continuous 5-FU before gemcitabine- or fluoropyrimidine-based chemodiation is also recommended as an adjuvant treatment, with subsequent chemotherapy being an option (NCCN, 2017).

In the advanced or metastatic setting, approved chemotherapy regimens are FOLFIRINOX (infusion and bolus 5-FU, oxaliplatin, irinotecan, and folinic acid); gemcitabine monotherapy; gemcitabine plus nab-paclitaxel; gemcitabine plus erlotinib; gemcitabine plus cisplatin (in *BRCA* and *PALB2* mutations); gemcitabine plus capecitabine; 5-FU, leucovorin, and nanoliposomal irinotecan; 5-FU, leucovorin, and oxaliplatin; FOLFOX (infusion and bolus 5-FU, folinic acid, and oxaliplatin); CAPOX (capecitabine and oxaliplatin); and continuous infusion 5-FU.

Depending on the initial regimen, performance status, and level of myelosuppression, a different regimen can be chosen as a second-line treatment. Clinical trials should always be considered in this population because of the lack of approved regimens and the small benefits seen in survival from the standard-of-care treatments.

The main areas where nursing can have an impact are early assessment of side effects and symptom management. Particularly with the aforementioned regimens, patients with pancreatic cancer commonly experience peripheral neuropathy, diarrhea, and myelosuppression (Lau & Cheung, 2017). Some patients may not understand the rationale for delaying treatment and may believe that this will cause detriment to their response. A thorough discussion of this topic may ease the anxiety of missing a treatment. Nurses should consider supportive care measures to assist patients in continuing treatment.

Radiation Therapy

Radiation can have benefits in the adjuvant or advanced setting. To date, no studies have demonstrated superiority of giving chemoradiation before versus after chemotherapy in the adjuvant setting (NCCN, 2017). Different radiation techniques are used in patients with pancreatic cancer. Because of the complex anatomy and surrounding organs, the goal is to preserve surrounding tissue and anatomy with minimal complications and toxicity. Intensity-modulated radiation therapy, stereotactic body radiation therapy, and three-dimensional conformal radiation therapy are used in this population (NCCN, 2017). Stereotactic body radiation therapy should be avoided if direct invasion of the bowel or stomach is observed on CT, MRI, or endoscopy (NCCN, 2017). According to NCCN (2017) guidelines, recommendations for radiation therapy are typically made based on several clinical scenarios: resectable/borderline, resectable in the neoadjuvant setting, locally advanced/unresectable, adjuvant setting after surgical resection, palliative radiation therapy, and in the recurrent setting. This may or may not include a chemosensitizing agent.

Nursing care for patients undergoing radiation therapy includes providing education about the timing of radiation and the different phases of preparation (planning and simulation) prior to starting treatment. The time leading up to treatment may be prolonged depending on surgical recovery. Oncology nurses should also be advocates for patients before, during, and after treatment because patients will be seen more frequently in the radiation therapy clinic. Communication between the radiation oncologist and medical oncologist should be open if side effects arise and supportive care is required. When adding chemotherapy to radiation, the risk of side effects such as diarrhea, mucositis, and myelosuppression may increase (Lau & Cheung, 2017). Providing detailed education on potential side effects and whom to contact will also allow patients to feel supported through treatment, especially if the treatment is for curative intent.

Immunotherapy

Immunotherapy is making an impact in many various cancers; however, an impact in pancreatic cancer has not yet been seen. Clinical trials in this area are ongoing.

Guidelines for Treatment

It is estimated that by 2030, approximately 70% of all cancers will be diagnosed in adults aged 65 years or older (Smith, Smith, Hurria, Hortobagyi, & Buchholz, 2009). According to ACS (2016), the risk of developing pancreatic cancer increases with age. Almost all patients are older than age 45 years, and approximately two-thirds are at least 65 years old. The average age at diagnosis of pancreatic cancer is 71 years (ACS, 2016). As a result, pancreatic cancer is a disease of the older adult, with the small exception of those patients who may have a familial history. NCCN does not have specific guidelines related to the care of older adults with pancreatic cancer as it does with colon, rectal, and hepatocellular carcinoma. However, it focuses on ensuring completion of a comprehensive geriatric assessment for older adults. The assessment includes functional status, comorbidities, cognitive function, nutritional status, polypharmacy, medication review, psychological status, and social support (NCCN, 2017). As a result, the focus should not be on age but on functional status. This should be considered with all types of treatments for pancreatic cancer (surgery, chemotherapy, and radiation).

Clinical Trials

Clinical trials are ongoing for every stage of pancreatic cancer, including many in the adjuvant setting and the advanced and metastatic setting. Current lists of trials are available at the ClinicalTrials.gov website (https://clinicaltrials.gov) and national pancreatic cancer advocacy group websites. Currently, three promising trials in pancreatic cancer are ongoing: the ALLIANCE trial in the neoadjuvant setting, a Radiation Therapy Oncology Group trial in the adjuvant setting, and a trial using napabucasin (a stemness inhibitor identified by its ability to inhibit STAT3-driven gene transcription and spherogenesis of cancer stem cells) in metastatic pancreatic cancer.

Much of the emphasis in clinical trial research is on precision medicine. Many institutions, companies, and national organizations are collaborating to identify specific markers in tumors to be able to ultimately match that marker with a treatment-specific drug or regimen. Ultimately, the goal is to show improvement in outcomes and decrease in side effects. Additionally, much effort is being placed on data sharing so that patients can be informed of clinical trials that are tailored to the specifics of their tumor. As a result of clinical trial research and advancements in technology, the current age of treatment is advancing.

Nursing Care

Patients diagnosed with pancreatic cancer have significant physical and emotional challenges because of the dismal prognosis and limited treatment options. The type of patient and family support varies as the disease progresses. However, from diagnosis to the end of treatment, focus should be provided on quality of life. This includes but is not limited to symptom management and supportive care services that will enhance the treatment experience to achieve better outcomes. The nursing role in the treatment of patients with pancreatic cancer should also focus on patient education and advocacy. Communication is key to helping patients understand the rationale for treatment interventions, and developing rapport with patients will provide an avenue to discuss side effects, including physical, emotional, and psychosocial issues, as they arise. Early management of symptoms will ultimately improve patient outcomes and quality of life and avoid unnecessary hospital admissions. Understanding the disease process and keeping up to date with the latest treatment options will equip oncology nurses with the tools necessary to provide quality care for this patient population.

Prognosis

Similar to the incidence and mortality rates for pancreatic cancer, the prognosis is poor, despite curative intent. According to ACS (2018), for all stages combined, the five-year survival rate is 8%. When broken down further, the five-year survival rate is 32% for localized disease and 3% for metastatic disease. As a result, systemic treatment is recommended to improve these low numbers, depending on patient clinical characteristics.

Prevention

Guidelines related to prevention of pancreatic cancer have not been established. The areas where prevention is addressed are in patients with confirmed genetic predispositions related to high-risk syndromes or mutations.

Patients with genetic syndromes associated with higher risk for pancreatic cancer should be considered for genetic testing as mentioned previously (see Risk Factors). In particular, patients with a family history of pancreatitis, melanoma, and cancers of the pancreas, colorectum, breast, and ovaries should be evaluated (NCCN, 2017). Patients of Ashkenazi Jewish ancestry and those who are young (age 50 years or younger) should also be referred for genetic counseling.

Surveillance

In patients who have undergone resection for pancreatic cancer, NCCN (2017) recommends a history and physical examination for symptom assessment every 3–6 months for two years, then every 6–12 months. Use of CA 19-9 and CT scans every three to six months for two years after surgical resection is lower in evidence and classified as a category 2A. However, because of the high risk of recurrence during the first year after completion of treatment, many providers will use imaging and laboratory studies to assist in the management of these patients.

Survivorship

Although survivorship programs have existed for many years, it recently has been a rising topic in the forefront of post-treatment care, with many institutions having to meet requirements that ensure survivorship care is provided. However, it is difficult to discuss survivorship with patients with pancreatic cancer who have a very high risk of recurrence even after curative intent. As a result, a structured survivorship program is lacking. NCI states that an individual is a cancer survivor from the time of diagnosis, through the balance of his or her life (NCI Office of Cancer Survivorship, 2014). Family members, friends, and caregivers are also affected by the survivorship experience and therefore are included in this definition (NCI Office of Cancer Survivorship, 2014). Physicians and advanced practice providers should be cautious when presenting survivorship to patients with pancreatic cancer. Patients should be educated on the purpose of survivorship care because this can cause heightened expectations regarding survival. Despite the dismal numbers in this disease, patients should be educated after treatment on important survivorship issues, including late effects of treatment (particularly peripheral neuropathy) and surveillance. Another area identified as critical to address in this population is depression. Depression was found in 33%–70% of patients with pancreatic cancer (Torgerson & Wiebe, 2013). Being able to identify patients with depression and provide them the support (referral to psychosocial services) and tools they need will allow a better quality of life after treatment.

Preventive strategies, such as increasing physical activity and maintaining a healthy weight to decrease recurrence risk, are important talking points in health education. Additionally, having a primary care physician available to care for the routine medical problems that may arise after treatment is critical to the continued care of cancer survivors. For nurses and providers, maintaining communication with the entire care team regarding post-treatment care will assist in having good communication pathways that will benefit patients' survival and quality of life.

Summary

Pancreatic cancer continues to be difficult to prevent and treat. However, more available options have evolved over recent years. Awareness of pancreatic cancer and advocacy in providing funding for clinical trials dedicated to studying and treating pancreatic cancer have also increased.

Surgery continues to be the only curative option, and risk of recurrence is high. As a result, more clinical trials in the adjuvant and neoadjuvant setting are evolving to reduce this risk. Additionally, the role of immunotherapy and other targeted agents is being studied within the arena of precision medicine in many stages of pancreatic cancer.

Patients with pancreatic cancer are very complex, and an interprofessional approach should be taken when treating these patients. The role of the nurse in the interprofessional team is one of an educator and patient advocate. It also entails supporting patients, family members, and caregivers through treatment by providing education on symptom management and the benefits of palliative care.

References

American Cancer Society. (2016). Pancreatic cancer risk factors. Retrieved from https://www.cancer.org/cancer/pancreatic-cancer/causes-risks-prevention/risk-factors.html

American Cancer Society. (2018). *Cancer facts and figures 2018*. Atlanta, GA: Author.

Ansari, D., Ansari, D., Andersson, R., & Andrén-Sandberg, Å. (2015). Pancreatic cancer and thromboembolic disease, 150 years after Trousseau. *Hepatobiliary Surgery and Nutrition, 4*, 325–335. https://doi.org/10.3978/j.issn.2304-3881.2015.06.08

Aşkan, G., Bağci, P., Memiş, B., & Baştürk, O. (2017). Intraductal neoplasms of the pancreas: An update. *Turkish Journal of Pathology, 33*, 87–102. https://doi.org/10.5146/tjpath.2017.01386

Conroy, T., Bachet, J.B., Ayav, A., Huguet, F., Lambert, A., Caramella, C., ... Ducreux, M. (2016). Current standards and new innovative approaches for treatment of pancreatic cancer. *European Journal of Cancer, 57*, 10–22. https://doi.org/10.1016/j.ejca.2015.12.026

Ferlay, J., Soerjomataram, I., Dikshit, R., Eser, D., Mathers, C., Rebelo, M., ... Bray, F. (2015). Cancer incidence and mortality worldwide: Sources, methods and major patterns in GLOBOCAN 2012. *International Journal of Cancer, 136*, E359–E386. https://doi.org/10.1002/ijc.29210

Hruban, R.H., Canto, M.I., Goggins, M., Schulick, R., & Klein, A.P. (2010). Update on familial pancreatic cancer. *Advances in Surgery, 44*, 293–311. https://doi.org/10.1016/j.yasu.2010.05.011

International Agency for Research on Cancer. (n.d.). GLOBOCAN 2012: Estimated cancer incidence, mortality and prevalence worldwide in 2012. Retrieved from http://publications.iarc.fr/Databases/Iarc-Cancerbases/GLOBOCAN-2012-Estimated-Cancer-Incidence-Mortality-And-Prevalence-Worldwide-In-2012-V1.0-2012

Kakar, S., Pawlik, T.M., Allen, P.J., & Vauthey, J.-N. (2017). Exocrine pancreas. In M.B. Amin (Ed.), *AJCC cancer staging manual* (8th ed., pp. 337–347). Chicago, IL: Springer.

Krantz, B.A., Yu, K.H., & O'Reilly, E.M. (2017). Pancreas adenocarcinoma: Novel therapeutics. *Chinese Clinical Oncology, 6*(3), 30. https://doi.org/10.21037/cco.2017.06.14

Larssen, L., Medhus, A.W., & Hauge, T. (2009). Treatment of malignant gastric outlet obstruction with stents: An evaluation of the reported variables for clinical outcome. *BMC Gastroenterology, 9*, 45. https://doi.org/10.1186/1471-230X-9-45

Lau, S.C., & Cheung, W.Y. (2017). Evolving treatment landscape for early and advanced pancreatic cancer. *World Journal of Gastrointestinal Oncology, 9*, 281–292. https://doi.org/10.4251/wjgo.v9.i7.281

Lowery, M.A., Jordan, E.J., Basturk, O., Ptashkin, R.N., Zehir, A., Berger, M.F., ... O'Reilly, E.M. (2017). Real-time genomic profiling of pancreatic ductal adenocarcinoma: Potential actionability and correlation with clinical phenotype. *Clinical Cancer Research, 23*, 6094–6100. https://doi.org/10.1158/1078-0432.CCR-17-0899

National Cancer Institute. (n.d.). Pancreatic cancer. In *NCI dictionary of cancer terms*. Retrieved from https://www.cancer.gov/publications/dictionaries/cancer-terms?CdrID=44521

National Cancer Institute. (2018, May 24). Pancreatic cancer treatment (PDQ®) [Health professional version]. Retrieved from https://www.cancer.gov/types/pancreatic/hp/pancreatic-treatment-pdq

National Cancer Institute Office of Cancer Survivorship. (2014, May 30). Definitions. Retrieved from https://www.cancercontrol.cancer.gov/ocs/statistics/definitions.html

National Comprehensive Cancer Network. (2017). *NCCN Framework for Resource Stratification of NCCN Guidelines (NCCN Framework™): Pancreatic adenocarcinoma: Basic resources* [v.3.2017]. Retrieved from https://www.nccn.org/professionals/physician_gls/pdf/pancreatic_basic.pdf

Neoptolemos, J.P., Palmer, D.H., Ghaneh, P., Psarelli, E.E., Valle, J.W., Halloran, C.M., ... Büchler, M.W. (2017). Comparison of adjuvant gemcitabine and capecitabine with gemcitabine monotherapy in patients with resected pancreatic (ESPAC-4): A multicentre, open-label, randomised, phase 3 trial. *Lancet, 389,* 1011–1024. https://doi.org/10.1016/S0140-6736(16)32409-6

Pagliari, D., Saviano, A., Serricchio, M.L., Dal Lago, A.A., Brizi, M.G., Lanza, F., ... Attili, F. (2017). Uptodate in the assessment and management of intraductal papillary mucinous neoplasms of the pancreas. *European Review for Medical and Pharmacological Sciences, 21,* 2858–2874. Retrieved from https://www.europeanreview.org/article/12946

Seicean, A. (2014). Celiac plexus neurolysis in pancreatic cancer: The endoscopic ultrasound approach. *World Journal of Gastroenterology, 20,* 110–117. https://doi.org/10.3748/wjg.v20.i1.110

Simoes, P.K., Olson, S.H., Saldia, A., & Kurtz, R.C. (2017). Epidemiology of pancreatic adenocarcinoma. *Chinese Clinical Oncology, 6*(3), 24. https://doi.org/10.21037/cco.2017.06.32

Smith, B.D., Smith, G.L., Hurria, A., Hortobagyi, G.N., & Buchholz, T.A. (2009). Future of cancer incidence in the United States: Burdens upon an aging, changing nation. *Journal of Clinical Oncology, 27,* 2758–2765. https://doi.org/10.1200/JCO.2008.20.8983

Toft, J., Hadden, W.J., Laurence, J.M., Lam, V., Yuen, L., Janssen, A., & Pleass, H. (2017). Imaging modalities in the diagnosis of pancreatic adenocarcinoma: A systematic review and meta-analysis of sensitivity, specificity and diagnostic accuracy. *European Journal of Radiology, 92,* 17–23. https://doi.org/10.1016/j.ejrad.2017.04.009

Torgerson, S., & Wiebe, L.A. (2013). Supportive care of the patient with advanced pancreatic cancer. *Oncology, 27,* 183–190. Retrieved from http://www.cancernetwork.com/pancreatic-cancer/supportive-care-patient-advanced-pancreatic-cancer

Walters, D.M., LaPar, D.J., de Lange, E.E., Sarti, M., Stokes, J.B., Adams, R.B., & Bauer, T.W. (2011). Pancreas-protocol imaging at a high-volume center leads to improved preoperative staging of pancreatic ductal adenocarcinoma. *Annals of Surgical Oncology, 18,* 2764–2771. https://doi.org/10.1245/s10434-011-1693-4

CHAPTER 5

Neuroendocrine Cancers

Pamela Ryan, BSN, RN, ONN-CG, and Brianne Voros, MS

Introduction

Neuroendocrine tumors (NETs) are a rare group of neoplasms that derive from neuroendocrine cells of the neuroendocrine system present throughout the entire body. Although most often found in the gastroenteropancreatic and bronchopulmonary tracts, NETs can originate almost anywhere in the body and differ in biologic behavior depending on the primary tumor site (the anatomic site that produced the first tumor). NETs are characterized by their ability to hypersecrete hormones, resulting in various clinical presentations. Symptoms from excess hormone production complicate the diagnosis of NETs because these symptoms can also be attributed to other common diseases, such as irritable bowel syndrome, Crohn disease, or menopause (Vinik & Chaya, 2016). Because of the variable and nonspecific clinical presentation, clinicians may not consider NETs in their differential diagnosis. Most patients may undergo evaluation by multiple physicians and centers before reaching the final diagnosis of NET.

Historically, NETs were referred to as carcinoids after Siegfried Oberndorfer used the term *karzinoide,* or "carcinoma-like," to describe their appearance (Modlin et al., 2008). His belief was that these slow-growing tumors were benign (Modlin et al., 2008). However, as these tumors were studied in more depth, it became clear that not all carcinoids demonstrated the same behavior. In 1963, Williams and Sandler proposed a classification system to distinguish NETs by embryonic origin and related these groups to histologic behavior and clinical presentation. They subdivided NETs into three groups: foregut, midgut, and hindgut. Tumors of the stomach, duodenum, pancreas, bronchus, and lung were referred to as foregut carcinoids. Tumors of the small intestine, cecum, proximal colon, and appendix were referred to as midgut carcinoids. Tumors of the distal colon and rectum were referred to as hindgut carcinoids (Modlin, Kidd, Latich, Zikusoka, & Shapiro, 2005). Although this classification system was the first to relate primary site with clinicopathologic differences in NETs, the lack of usefulness and clinical relevance limited the adoption of this system by clinicians. In 1980, the World Health Organization used the term *carcinoid* to refer to most NETs and further subdivided carcinoid tumors into enterochromaffin cells, gastrin cells, and an undefined group. This terminology was confusing, as it was used in different contexts by clinicians and pathologists. Thus, in 2000 and again in 2010, the World Health Organization updated its classification system to provide clarity on nomenclature. As understanding of the behavior of NETs improved, numerous systems of classification were proposed. Currently, guidelines for classification include anatomic site as the primary component (Chen, Yi, & He, 2013).

Bronchial and gastrointestinal NETs are often referred to as carcinoids, whereas pancreatic NETs (PNETs) are referred to as islet cell tumors. NETs can be broadly subdivided based on functional status. NETs that present with a clinical syndrome associated with symptoms of excess hormone production are referred to as functional, and NETs that lack classic symptoms and may be completely silent are referred to as nonfunctional (Díez, Teulé, & Salazar, 2013).

Incidence and Epidemiology

Because of the rare and slow-growing nature of NETs, early studies evaluating the epidemiology of these tumors are limited. The most comprehensive analyses to date include large, population-based registry studies with significant long-term follow-up. Previous studies suggest that the incidence and prevalence of NETs are rising, but the cause of this increase is unclear. With increased awareness among physicians and improvements in detection methods, such as computed tomography (CT) and endoscopy, the increased incidence is likely associated with increased detection of NETs at early disease stages (Modlin et al., 2008; Yao et al., 2008).

In 2008, Yao et al. analyzed epidemiology, as well as other prognostic factors in NETs, in 35,825 patients identified in the Surveillance, Epidemiology, and End Results (SEER) database. Annual age-adjusted incidence of NETs in all sites significantly increased from 1.09 per 100,000 people in 1973 to 5.25 per 100,000 in 2004 (Yao et al., 2008). In a recent retrospective, population-based study of 64,971 patients with NETs from the SEER database, the annual age-adjusted incidence of NETs in the United States was calculated to be 6.98 per 100,000 people, with an estimated prevalence of 171,321 patients affected with NETs as of January 1, 2014 (Dasari et al., 2017). Lung NETs are the second most common lung cancer after squamous carcinomas, and gastrointestinal NETs are the second most common gastrointestinal cancer after colon cancer (Dasari et al., 2017).

Etiology and Risk Factors

The etiology of NETs of all primary sites is unknown. Enterochromaffin cells, also known as Kulchitsky cells, are present in the lumen of the digestive tract and regulate gastrointestinal activity, specifically intestinal motility and secretion. These cells are thought to give rise to carcinoid tumors (Modlin et al., 2008).

Somatostatin is a peptide hormone that inhibits the secretion of several hormones, including growth hormone, thyroid-stimulating hormone, insulin, glucagon, serotonin, and gastrin, by binding to the cell surface of its target. The function of somatostatin is mediated by its binding to a family of G-protein–coupled receptors, termed *somatostatin receptors* (SSTRs), of which five subtypes have been characterized (SSTR1–5). NETs have been found to overexpress SSTRs on their surface and vary in frequency of overexpression of each SSTR subtype based on their tissue of origin (Maxwell & Howe, 2015). The overexpression of SSTRs by NETs allows for the targeting of these receptors using imaging with radiolabeled somatostatin analogs (SSAs) and therapy with somatostatin synthetic analogs (octreotide) that bind to the SSTRs (Maxwell & Howe, 2015).

Because the underlying cause of NETs is unknown, no preventable risk factors have been identified. However, multiple factors have been associated with an increased risk for developing a NET. Most notably, a family history of multiple endocrine neoplasia type 1 (MEN1) has been associated with gastroenteropancreatic NETs (Ramage et al., 2012). The incidence of MEN1 in gastroenteropancreatic NETs is 5%–30% and varies significantly at different anatomic sites (Ramage et al., 2012). Chronic use of proton pump inhibitors has shown a correlation in the risk of developing gastric NETs, probably caused by reflex hypergastrinemia (Helgadóttir, Metz, Yang, Rhim, & Björnsson, 2014; Raines et al., 2014).

Signs and Symptoms

Clinical Presentation

Clinical presentation of patients with NETs is dependent on multiple factors, including location of the primary tumor, functional status (hormone production), and extent of disease (Modlin et al., 2008). Functional status is a unique aspect of NETs, causing symptoms that vary based on the type of hormone they produce. NETs that secrete hormones and produce a clinical syndrome are referred to as functional, whereas most NETs are nonfunctional and present with symptoms associated with nonspecific, mechanical complications of tumor burden. Typically, functional NETs are named for the hormone they produce. A variety of clinical syndromes result from these hormones, including carcinoid syndrome, Zollinger-Ellison syndrome, and Sweet syndrome. Carcinoid syndrome is present in less than 10% of patients with carcinoid NETs and occurs more frequently in tumors of the ileum, jejunum, and lung that have metastasized to the liver (Vinik & Chaya, 2016). Only 30%–40% of NETs are functional (Vinik & Chaya, 2016). In nonfunctional NETs, which have a silent clinical presentation, the majority of patients present with symptoms resulting from mass effects (Vinik & Chaya, 2016).

Unfortunately, diagnosis of metastatic NETs often occurs late with the onset of symptoms of carcinoid syndrome (Woltering, Vinik, O'Dorisio, Go, & Mamikunian, 2012). Clinical presentation complicated by nonspecific and variable symptoms by NETs of different primary sites often leads to a delay in diagnosis by an average of 7–10 years (Singh et al., 2017). Because of the high metastatic potential of NETs combined with delayed diagnosis, 58% of patients present with metastatic disease at the time of diagnosis (Singh et al., 2017). Regardless of the primary site of origin, the liver is the most common location of metastatic disease. Metastatic disease in the liver may be the only identifiable NET disease in symptomatic patients. Metastatic NETs in the liver also have the ability to secrete hormones and may be the primary source of symptoms in these patients. Liver metastatic NETs have been shown to be a prognostic indicator of poor survival regardless of primary tumor site (Maxwell, Sherman, O'Dorisio, Bellizzi, & Howe, 2016).

The hallmark clinical presentation in functional NETs is a combination of vague, nonspecific symptoms resulting from the hypersecretion of certain hormones or substances (Vinik et al., 2010). Obtaining a detailed history and characterization of each symptom from patients is important for clinicians to rule out symptoms that may be associated with other disease processes. Functional NETs that secrete serotonin produce symptoms such as cutaneous flushing, intermittent abdominal pain, diarrhea, tachycardia, wheezing, or asthma-like symptoms. Collectively, these symptoms constitute the clinical presentation referred to as carcinoid syndrome (Vinik et al., 2010).

Flushing is the sudden onset of red or purple coloration and warmth of the skin of the face or neck and is one of the most common symptoms associated with NETs (Vinik et al., 2010). NET-related flushing is described as dry, intermittent flushing lasting one to five minutes, whereas constant flushing or sweating is typically attributed to a cardiovascular or menopausal source (Vinik et al., 2010).

Diarrhea in patients with suspected NETs is more difficult to differentiate from other conditions. Comparison of the frequency and characteristics of the diarrhea can be important in ruling out other causes, such as irritable bowel syndrome, hypokalemia, laxative abuse, and acidosis syndrome (Vinik & Chaya, 2016).

Functional NETs may secrete other peptide hormones, such as insulin, vasoactive intestinal peptide (VIP), glucagon, or gastrin, that can be distinguished by the various clinical syndromes manifesting with nonspecific symptoms, such as hypoglycemia, hypergastrinemia, severe diarrhea, dehydration, or a migratory rash. Table 5-1 summarizes the types of NETs, the clinical syndromes they produce, and common symptoms in clinical presentation.

Nonfunctional NETs may be associated with intermittent abdominal pain, cramping, jaundice, weight loss, or nausea due to mass effects. Mass effects are caused by tumor growth or gross tumor size affecting the normal function of nearby vital organs, structures, or blood vessels. For example, NET metastases in the abdomen may grow to encase the vasculature that supplies blood to the bowel. Partial or complete encasement of the mesenteric vasculature may result in intestinal ischemia and manifest as intestinal angina (Vinik & Chaya, 2016).

Foregut Neuroendocrine Tumors

Stomach

NETs can be categorized based on embryologic site of origin: foregut (lung, stomach, duodenum, and pancreas), midgut (jejunum, ileum, appendix, and cecum), and hindgut (transverse colon, descending colon, and rectum). NETs of the stomach are often referred to as gastric carcinoids or gastric NETs. Three types of gastric NETs can be distinguished based on clinical and biochemical characteristics.

Type 1 gastric NETs often present as multiple small lesions and are considered relatively nonaggressive. Patients present with atrophic gastritis, low gastric acid production, high serum gastrin levels, and pernicious anemia as a result of autoimmune gastritis. High gastrin levels stimulate carcinoid tumor growth in the stomach (Vinik & Chaya, 2016).

Type 2 gastric NETs are associated with Zollinger-Ellison syndrome and also may present as multiple small, nonaggressive lesions. Zollinger-Ellison syndrome manifests as frequent or recurrent peptic ulcers due to excess gastric acid production and high serum gastrin lev-

Table 5-1. Neuroendocrine Origin, Primary Tumor, Clinical Syndrome, Hormones, and Presentation

Embryologic Origin	Foregut								Midgut	Midgut and Hindgut
Primary Tumor	Stomach			Pancreas					Duodenum	Intestinal NETs and Rectal
Type of NET	Type 1 Gastric NETs	Type 2 Gastric NETs	Type 3 Gastric NETs	Insulinoma	Glucagonoma	VIPoma	Somatostatinoma		Gastrinoma	Carcinoids
Clinical syndrome	Pernicious anemia	Zollinger-Ellison syndrome	Atypical carcinoid syndrome	Whipple triad	Sweet syndrome	Verner-Morrison syndrome	—		Zollinger-Ellison syndrome	Carcinoid syndrome
Associated hormones	Gastrin	Gastrin, pancreastatin	—	Insulin, proinsulin, C-peptide	Glucagon	Vasoactive intestinal polypeptide	Somatostatin		Gastrin	Serotonin

(Continued on next page)

Table 5-1. Neuroendocrine Origin, Primary Tumor, Clinical Syndrome, Hormones, and Presentation *(Continued)*

Embryologic Origin	Foregut							Midgut	Midgut and Hindgut
Primary Tumor	Stomach			Pancreas				Duodenum	Intestinal NETs and Rectal
Type of NET	Type 1 Gastric NETs	Type 2 Gastric NETs	Type 3 Gastric NETs	Insulinoma	Glucagonoma	VIPoma	Somatostatinoma	Gastrinoma	Carcinoids
Clinical presentation	Autoimmune gastritis and pernicious anemia, decreased gastric acid, diarrhea, increased serum gastrin	Diarrhea, increased gastric acid, increased serum gastrin, peptic ulcers, steatorrhea	Cherry red, patchy flushing; normal serum gastrin and gastric acid	Confusion, dizziness, hypoglycemia, sweating	Diarrhea, flushing, glucose intolerance, necrotizing migratory rash, weight loss	Diarrhea, dehydration, hypercalcemia, hypokalemia	Anemia, cholelithiasis, diabetes mellitus, steatorrhea, weight loss	Abdominal pain, recurrent peptic ulcers, secretory diarrhea, steatorrhea	Cutaneous flushing, diarrhea, gastrointestinal bleeding, intermittent abdominal pain, tachycardia, wheezing or asthma-like symptoms

NET—neuroendocrine tumor; VIP—vasoactive intestinal peptide
Note. Based on information from Vinik & Chaya, 2016.

els (Vinik & Chaya, 2016). The tumors in the stomach grow as a result of excess gastrin produced by an islet cell tumor of the pancreas (Maxwell, O'Dorisio, & Howe, 2016).

Type 3 gastric NETs are spontaneous solitary tumors that often are larger than type 1 and type 2 tumors. Clinical presentation of type 3 gastric NETs may be associated with normal gastrin and gastric acid levels. Associated with a high tendency to metastasize, type 3 gastric NETs typically exhibit very aggressive behavior and are the type most likely to cause tumor-related deaths (Vinik & Chaya, 2016).

Pancreas

PNETs are thought to derive from pancreatic islet cells, also called islets of Langerhans, and are collectively referred to as islet cell tumors. While the majority of PNETs are silent (nonfunctional), functional PNETs are named for the hormone they secrete (Vinik & Chaya, 2016).

Insulinomas are the most common type of functional PNET. These tumors often are small and difficult to find but can produce severe and life-threatening symptoms. The symptoms resulting from insulinomas, collectively known as the Whipple triad, can include headache, blurred vision, seizures, confusion, dizziness, or weakness and may lead to unconsciousness or coma, all due to hypoglycemia (Maxwell, O'Dorisio, & Howe, 2016). Demonstration of Whipple triad symptoms is highly suggestive of an insulinoma. Diagnosis may be confirmed by the presence of increased insulin levels during a 72-hour fast (Maxwell, O'Dorisio, & Howe, 2016; Vinik & Chaya, 2016).

Gastrinomas are named for their hypersecretion of the peptide hormone gastrin and can be associated with Zollinger-Ellison syndrome. They account for 15% of all functional PNETs (Maxwell, O'Dorisio, & Howe, 2016).

Glucagonomas are among the rarest of functional PNETs and are estimated to be less than 1% of cases (Maxwell, O'Dorisio, & Howe, 2016). Classic presentation of patients with these tumors includes necrolytic migratory erythema (red, blistering rash that eventually crusts and fluctuates in severity), deep vein thrombosis, diabetes mellitus, stomatitis (inflamed and sore mouth), and diarrhea (Maxwell, O'Dorisio, & Howe, 2016; Vinik & Chaya, 2016).

VIPomas are named for their hypersecretion of VIP and represent less than 2% of functional PNET cases (Maxwell, O'Dorisio, & Howe, 2016). Clinical presentation due to elevated VIP levels is referred to as Verner-Morrison syndrome. This syndrome is characterized by profuse, watery diarrhea; marked hypokalemia; and dehydration. Patients may have 10–20 watery stools per day and can experience potentially lethal electrolyte disturbances (Vinik & Chaya, 2016).

Somatostatinomas are extremely rare functional PNETs that account for less than 1% of all PNETs (Maxwell, O'Dorisio, & Howe, 2016). Hypersecretion of somatostatin by these tumors causes gastroparesis, constipation, and crampy abdominal pain (Maxwell, O'Dorisio, & Howe, 2016).

Nonfunctional PNETs represent approximately 70%–80% of all PNETs and usually present with symptoms due to mass effect (Vinik & Chaya, 2016). Patients with nonfunctional PNETs often present with obstruction of the bile duct or portal vein; splenic vein occlusion, which causes gastric varices and hypersplenism; or abdominal pain due to invasion of the abdominal vasculature and retroperitoneal nerves (Boudreaux, 2011). They are commonly metastatic at the time of diagnosis (Vinik & Chaya, 2016).

Duodenum

Duodenal NETs are most often silent (nonfunctional). However, functional duodenal NETs hypersecrete gastrin, also producing Zollinger-Ellison syndrome, and can be difficult to distinguish from other pancreatic islet cell NETs.

Midgut Neuroendocrine Tumors: Jejunum, Ileum, Appendix, and Cecum

The majority (approximately 60%) of NETs originating in the jejunum, ileum, appendix, and cecum are silent, with no symptoms present (Ramage et al., 2012). Clinical presentation may include abdominal pain due to intermittent partial or complete bowel obstruction or intussusception, cramping, and gastrointestinal hemorrhage or melena (Boudreaux, 2011). Functional tumors hypersecrete serotonin, resulting in carcinoid syndrome. Classic carcinoid syndrome includes diarrhea, flushing, palpitations, and wheezing. Unfortunately, patients who present with some or all symptoms of carcinoid syndrome are likely to have metastatic disease to the liver at diagnosis (Vinik & Chaya, 2016). Bulky lymph node metastasis surrounding abdominal vessels also can cause intestinal ischemia, intestinal angina, and obstruction (Boudreaux et al., 2014).

Hindgut Neuroendocrine Tumors: Distal Colon and Rectum

NETs of the distal colon and rectum usually are silent and often found incidentally during routine colonoscopy (Vinik & Chaya, 2016). Typically, NETs of the distal colon and rectum are smaller tumors and less likely to metastasize. Larger tumors of this type usually are metastatic at diagnosis. Symptoms resulting from NETs of the colon and rectum include bleeding or rectal pain due to mass effects (Howe et al., 2017).

Diagnostic Evaluation

Diagnostic workup of patients with suspected NETs is dependent on clinical presentation and can include biochemical evaluation, a variety of imaging modalities, and pathologic evaluation. Identification of the primary tumor and assessment of the extent of local and metastatic disease are critical components in treatment planning and management of patients with NETs. Recent advances in both anatomic and functional imaging modalities have led to earlier detection of these tumors and have ultimately contributed to improved long-term patient survival (Maxwell, O'Dorisio, & Howe, 2016).

Biochemical Evaluation

Biochemical evaluation is an essential component used in the diagnosis of patients with suspected or known NETs. NETs produce a wide variety of clinical syndromes resulting from the hypersecretion of hormones or other biologically active molecules. When patients present with vague or nonspecific symptoms that are also associated with other disease processes, functional or nonfunctional peptides specific to NETs (collectively referred to as biomarkers) can be detected in the blood or urine.

In patients with symptoms associated with carcinoid syndrome, biochemical evaluation involves detection of the biomarkers believed to be involved in the underlying mechanisms of the symptoms of carcinoid syndrome. Serotonin is thought to be the principal cause of diarrhea in carcinoid syndrome and can be detected in blood circulation (Woltering et al., 2012). A less invasive option involves detection of 5-hydroxyindoleacetic acid (5-HIAA), one of the main metabolites of serotonin, in urine. Nonfunctional secretory proteins, such as chromogranin A, neurokinin A, and pancreastatin, are also commonly used in biochemical evaluation and assessment of response to therapy (Woltering et al., 2012). Any of the functional islet cell hormones, when present, are also useful markers (Woltering et al., 2012).

In patients with symptoms of functional PNETs, biochemical evaluation depends on the clinical presentation and should include evaluation of hormones relevant to the suspected type of functional PNET (Vinik & Chaya, 2016).

Imaging Modalities

Surgical resection of the primary tumor and all metastatic disease is currently the only curative option for NETs. Overall survival is directly linked to completeness of resection of the primary tumor, as well as of hepatic and extrahepatic metastases. Thus, determining resectability preoperatively relies on visualization of disease with preoperative imaging (Boudreaux et al., 2014; Deppen et al., 2016; Maxwell, O'Dorisio, & Howe, 2016).

Computed Tomography

Often used as the initial diagnostic tool for evaluation of a patient with a suspected NET, CT is widely available at most institutions. A CT scan is routinely used with IV contrast for possible detection of the primary tumor, evaluation of the extent of local disease, and assessment for staging of locoregional and distant metastases. It can be obtained relatively quickly with high resolution and aids in resection planning (Maxwell, O'Dorisio, & Howe, 2016).

Magnetic Resonance Imaging

Magnetic resonance imaging (MRI) is an imaging modality that provides a cross-sectional image using a magnet. It has been shown to have increased sensitivity for detecting NET metastasis in the liver compared with CT scanning and often is used to evaluate patients with known or suspected metastatic disease in the liver (Maxwell, O'Dorisio, & Howe, 2016).

Functional Imaging Modalities

Standard imaging techniques, such as CT and MRI scans, are useful as initial studies, but they have no specificity for NETs and are plagued by false-positive and false-negative results (Maxwell, O'Dorisio, & Howe, 2016). Extent of resectability often is determined intraoperatively (Boudreaux et al., 2014).

In many types of cancer, traditional positron-emission tomography (PET) scans use the radiotracer 18-fluorodeoxyglucose (^{18}FDG), a radiolabeled glucose molecule, to evaluate patients for metastatic disease. When rapidly dividing tumor cells metabolize ^{18}FDG (radioactive glucose), the radiotracer component remains in the tumor cell and can be visualized on PET scan (Maxwell, O'Dorisio, & Howe, 2016). The high metabolic activity in some cancers allows for uptake of ^{18}FDG by tumors that can subsequently be imaged. In contrast, the slow-growing nature of NETs limits their metabolic activity and uptake of ^{18}FDG. Although ^{18}FDG-PET scan occasionally may show uptake in patients with NETs exhibiting aggressive metabolic activity or proliferative characteristics, ^{18}FDG-PET scan has limited utility to detect NETs in the majority of patients (Vinik & Chaya, 2016).

Because a high proportion of NETs express SSTRs on their surface, these receptors provide an alternative target for imaging to effectively detect primary tumors and associated metastases (Maxwell, O'Dorisio, & Howe, 2016; Vinik & Chaya, 2016). SSAs bind to

SSTRs on the surface of NET cells. Although SSAs were initially developed and used for symptom control, radiolabeled SSAs bind to NETs, which then allows for imaging of tumors. As a result, the most commonly used and reliable imaging modalities for NETs are SSA-based imaging (Maxwell, O'Dorisio, & Howe, 2016; Vinik & Chaya, 2016). The two techniques currently used are SSTR scintigraphy and PET-CT with gallium.

Somatostatin Receptor Scintigraphy

SSTR scintigraphy using indium-111 (^{111}In) bound to the SSA octreotide is commonly referred to as an octreotide scan. This technique provides a whole body, noninvasive method for imaging of NETs. To undergo an octreotide scan, patients are first injected intravenously with ^{111}In-octreotide. At 4 and 24 hours after injection, a two-dimensional whole body image is obtained using a gamma camera (Ramage et al., 2012). At most institutions, octreotide scan is performed in combination with single photon emission CT (known as SPECT). This combined technique allows for three-dimensional reconstruction and further assessment of regions of interest. Until recently, octreotide scan was the gold-standard imaging modality available in the United States for NETs. Unfortunately, its sensitivity and resolution are inferior to the more advanced PET scans using radiolabeled SSAs that are now available (Maxwell & Howe, 2015).

Positron-Emission Tomography

The gallium scan is a combined PET-CT scan that uses an alternate radiotracer bound to an SSA, such as gallium-68 (^{68}Ga)-dotatate, to take advantage of the biologic behavior of NETs (Deppen et al., 2016; Vinik & Chaya, 2016). Although both octreotide scan and gallium scan use the same biologic principles, gallium scans provide a significantly greater resolution and sensitivity and improved tolerance for patients. PET-CT with ^{68}Ga-dotatate takes 90 minutes from time of injection to scan completion and yields superior results (Vinik & Chaya, 2016). Despite its recent approval in 2016 for use in the United States, PET scanning with ^{68}Ga-dotatate is not a new technology. Many studies from Europe, Asia, Latin America, and Australia attest to this modality being an excellent technique for staging of NETs (Vinik & Chaya, 2016).

Guidelines for Diagnostic Evaluation

For gastrointestinal NETs, the National Comprehensive Cancer Network® (NCCN®, 2018) guidelines for diagnostic evaluation recommend abdominal or pelvic multiphasic CT scan or MRI and suggest considering octreotide scan or gallium scan, colonoscopy, small bowel imaging (such as CT enterography or capsule endoscopy), chest CT scan, and biochemical evaluation using appropriate biomarkers. Biochemical evaluation should include chromogranin A and 24-hour urine or serum 5-HIAA (NCCN, 2018).

In addition, NCCN (2018) guidelines recommend diagnostic evaluation of functional PNETs with abdominal or pelvic multiphasic CT scan or MRI, serum pancreatic polypeptide, chromogranin A, and serum levels of hormones associated with the suspected or known PNET subtypes. Suggestions for additional evaluation include considering octreotide or gallium scan, endoscopic ultrasound, and other biochemical evaluation as clinically indicated.

Histology and Staging

Histology and Grade

Histologic classification of NETs is based on tumor differentiation and tumor grade. Together, differentiation and grade determine the clinical behavior of NETs. *Differentiation* refers to the extent that these neoplasms resemble their non-neoplastic counterparts. *Grade* refers to the growth rate of these tumors, or their biologic aggressiveness. A combination of grading and staging is used to determine the course of treatment required (Klimstra, Modlin, Coppola, Lloyd, & Suster, 2010; Turaga & Kvols, 2011). Also included in the grading systems for NETs are assessments of the proliferative behavior of the tumor. Most NETs exhibit slow proliferative growth characteristics, but some demonstrate rapid proliferation. *Mitotic index* refers to the number of mitoses per high-powered fields (Rindi et al., 2010). *Ki-67 proliferative index* refers to the percentage of dividing cells, or cellular proliferation (Rindi et al., 2010). Tumors with a high mitotic or Ki-67 index are associated with more aggressive behavior and rapid cell growth (Rindi et al., 2010). Table 5-2 shows a summary of the current nomenclature and criteria for grading (Rindi et al., 2010).

Interprofessional management has been shown to be the most beneficial approach when determining treatment option for NETs. Therefore, a complete pathology report is essential. According to NCCN (2018) guidelines, a NET pathology report should include, at the very least, tumor differentiation, mitotic rate, and Ki-67 index to allow clinicians to make well-informed treatment decisions. Standardized pathology templates developed by the College of American Pathologists provide clinicians with summarized pathology information and include the following for NETs: anatomic site, diagnosis, stage, tumor

Table 5-2. Nomenclature for Histologic Classification and Grading of Neuroendocrine Tumors

Characteristic	Low Grade (G1)	Intermediate Grade (G2)	High Grade (G3)
Ki-67 proliferative index	< 3%	3%–20%	> 20%
Mitotic index	< 2 mitoses/10 HPF	2–20 mitoses/10 HPF	> 20 mitoses/10 HPF
Tumor differentiation	Well differentiated	Well differentiated	Poorly differentiated
WHO (2010) classification	Neuroendocrine tumor, grade 1	Neuroendocrine tumor, grade 2	Neuroendocrine carcinoma, grade 3 (large or small cell)

HPF—high-powered fields; WHO—World Health Organization

Note. Based on information from Rindi et al., 2010.

differentiation, grade, Ki-67 proliferative index, mitotic index, prognostic factors such as necrosis or vascular invasion, and margin status (Rindi et al., 2010).

Clinical Staging

Cancer staging refers to the process used to determine the location of the disease and extent to which the disease has spread. Staging systems generally include the size of the primary tumor, invasion of adjacent organs or structures, regional lymph node involvement, and distant metastatic disease. For staging of NETs, NCCN (2018) recommends the American Joint Committee on Cancer (AJCC) tumor-node-metastasis (TNM) staging system. The TNM staging system evaluates three categories. The tumor (T) category evaluates the primary tumor and involves assignment to a T subgroup based on evaluation of the extent of primary tumor disease. The nodal (N) category evaluates disease at regional lymph nodes located close to the primary tumor. The metastasis (M) category includes assessment of distant metastatic disease. In the eighth edition of the *AJCC Cancer Staging Manual*, NETs are subdivided by primary site of origin for staging, which is a significant improvement to previous editions, which staged NETs with other cancer types of the same primary site (Amin, 2017). Using staging to describe the magnitude of the primary (original) tumor, as well as the extent of disease spread, allows clinicians to estimate prognosis and design individualized treatment plans for patients.

Treatment

Interprofessional Management

In the past decade, major progress has occurred in clinician awareness of this disease, as well as in the diagnosis and management of NETs. Although surgical resection remains the only potentially curative treatment, a multimodal approach combining surgery with other available treatments has been shown to be most effective in treating patients with NETs. Other treatments involved in this multimodal approach may include SSAs for reduction of symptoms, systemic therapies, and liver-directed therapies (Boudreaux et al., 2014). With the availability of a wide variety of therapies targeting NETs, evaluation and consideration of all treatment modalities to develop an individualized, comprehensive treatment plan for each patient requires coordinated management by a team of NET specialists. Presentation of each patient for discussion and recommendations at a designated NET tumor board is paramount and is dependent on multispecialty participation, including surgeons, medical oncologists, pathologists, interventional radiologists, nuclear medicine specialists, nutritionists, gastroenterologists, clinical trial coordinators, nurses, and other clinical staff (Woltering et al., 2017).

Somatostatin Analogs

SSAs are the mainstay of therapy for syndromic and nonsyndromic NETs of all primary sites and have been proved to decrease hormone production and slow progression of disease (Cives & Strosberg, 2015). The two available agents most commonly used in NETs are octreotide and lanreotide. Both are available as long-acting, monthly depot injections (Caplin et al., 2014; Cives & Strosberg, 2015; Rinke et al., 2009).

The normal function of somatostatin is to inhibit pancreatic hormones that stimulate control of production and excretion of pancreatic enzymes (Go, Srihari, & Burns, 2010). Pancreatic enzymes assist in digestion of fats, carbohydrates, and proteins. SSAs mimic the effects of natural somatostatin and cause pancreatic insufficiency in 30% of patients who take them (Go et al., 2010). Side effects of chronic SSA treatment result from pancreatic insufficiency and include steatorrhea (excess fat in stool), diarrhea, malabsorption, and nausea. However, these side effects can easily be controlled using pancreatic enzyme replacement therapy, which involves ingestion of capsules containing a mixture of pancreatic enzymes (Go et al., 2010). Another function of somatostatin includes inhibition of hepatic bile secretion and gallbladder emptying. In patients treated with SSAs, gallbladder dysfunction may result in the production of gallstones (Saif, Larson, Kaley, & Shaib, 2010). Because of the risk of gallbladder dysfunction associated with chronic SSA treatment, prophylactic cholecystectomy is recommended as standard of care for patients who are treated with SSAs (NCCN, 2018; Woltering et al., 2017).

Surgery

Indications for surgery include curative intent, symptom control, and palliation for prolongation of life, as well as focused debulking to increase effectiveness of potential adjunctive therapies. Low- and intermediate-grade, well-differentiated NETs are approached surgically, whereas high-grade, poorly differentiated NETs are targeted using chemotherapy (Boudreaux, 2011). Surgery is indicated for relief of obstruction, often occurring in the intestines, bile duct, or ureter. Debulking functional tumors decreases hormone production. Because liver failure is the leading cause of death in patients with metastatic disease, removal of hepatic tumors while conserving normal liver function is undertaken whenever feasible and has been shown to double survival (Boudreaux et al., 2014).

When disease is confined to a limited area without diffuse metastasis, surgery often can be performed with curative intent. When faced with bulky bilobar liver metastases, patients can undergo staged surgical resection with separate procedures to address each side of the liver. In the first procedure, one side of the patient's liver is extensively debulked, and the patient is given time to recover. Because these tumors are typically slow growing, the opposite side of the liver can be addressed later with limited risk of recurrence of the resected disease between procedures. Recent studies have shown a 57% survival rate at 20 years with aggressive surgery (Boudreaux et al., 2014; Woltering et al., 2017). The decision for operability needs to be made in the context of a NET center with experienced clinicians to see this survival difference (Boudreaux et al., 2014; Woltering et al., 2017).

Preoperative Management

Critical components of preoperative management of patients with NETs include management of symptoms, nutrition optimization, and cardiac evaluation for carcinoid heart disease. A thorough nutritional assessment is an essential step in preoperative evaluation. Patients often are malnourished because of malabsorption from diarrhea, partial or complete intestinal obstruction, or food avoidance due to abdominal pain resulting from bowel ischemia (Boudreaux, 2011). Subsequent initiation of a nutrition program and improvement in nutritional status prior to surgery are vital to reduce postoperative complications and improve overall outcome (Boudreaux, 2011).

Carcinoid heart disease is characterized by right-sided heart failure induced by the destruction of heart valves resulting from excessive serotonin levels and carcinoid syndrome (Connolly, 2001). An attempt to control excess hormone production in functional NETs should be undertaken preoperatively using SSAs to facilitate a smoother perioperative course. IV high-dose octreotide (250–500 mcg/hr) is used intraoperatively to prevent carcinoid crisis (vasomotor collapse) often induced by tumor manipulation and serotonin release (Boudreaux, 2011). The use of epinephrine and other vasoconstrictors should be avoided because these compounds act as neurotransmitters, causing massive serotonin release by the tumor that leads to catastrophic cardiovascular collapse, or carcinoid crisis (Woltering, Wright, et al., 2016).

Studies indicate that primary intestinal tumors should be removed to prevent obstruction (Boudreaux, 2011). In the case of PNETs, removal of the primary tumor may prevent splenic, portal, or biliary obstruction (Woltering et al., 2017).

Intraoperative Management

Intraoperative management should include the use of IV octreotide at 250–500 mcg/hr for prophylaxis against carcinoid crisis. Management also includes avoidance of vasopressors and low filling pressures during hepatic resection to avoid back-bleeding from the liver (Woltering, Wright, et al., 2016). Steroids and antihistamines also are used to minimize carcinoid crisis (Woltering, Wright, et al., 2016).

Tools and Techniques

Complete resection of the primary tumor and all associated metastatic disease in NETs provides a significant survival advantage. Surgeons must overcome a variety of intraoperative challenges in surgical resection of NETs, whether the intent of resection is curative, palliative, or staged. Complex operations may last 7–10 hours and involve multiple surgeons to accomplish adequate resection (Howe et al., 2017). Many tools and techniques are used to assist surgeons with intraoperative tumor detection and complete resection (Boudreaux et al., 2014; Woltering et al., 2017).

An intraoperative handheld gamma counter (Neoprobe®) is used to detect tumors after injection of a radioactive isotope–labeled SSA and allows for probe-directed dissection, much like a metal detector at the beach (Boudreaux, 2011).

Lymphatic mapping involves the injection of blue dye into the primary tumor to improve completeness and adequacy of resection. Depending on tumor location, lymphatic mapping may allow for sparing of the ileocecal valve. Ileocecal valve sparing is recommended especially for patients who are already challenged with diarrhea (Boudreaux, 2011).

Postoperative Management

Postoperatively, patients are gradually weaned off SSA infusions over a few days to avoid precipitation of carcinoid crisis (Woltering, Wright, et al., 2016). Hypotension in the postoperative period is managed with volume infusions and boluses of IV SSAs (Woltering, Wright, et al., 2016). Vasopressors are contraindicated (Woltering, Wright, et al., 2016).

Transplantation

Liver transplantation or, rarely, multivisceral transplantation, including the liver, pancreas, and intestines, may be recommended when all disease can be removed with removal of the affected organ or organs (Cives & Strosberg, 2017). Currently, the presence of bone metastasis is an absolute contraindication to transplantation (Cives & Strosberg, 2017).

Systemic Therapy

Chemotherapy

Cytotoxic chemotherapy regimens reserved for high-grade (G3) NETs include 5-fluorouracil with streptozotocin for high-grade islet cell PNETs and cisplatin in combination with etoposide for high-grade PNETs, bronchial NETs, and gastrointestinal NETs (Strosberg et al., 2011).

Cytotoxic chemotherapy is not recommended for low- or intermediate-grade NETs (Kunz et al., 2013). The combination of capecitabine and temozolomide (CAPTEM) is used to treat unresectable low-grade (G1) and intermediate-grade (G2) gastrointestinal, pancreatic, and bronchial NETs (Ramirez et al., 2016). These oral agents are well tolerated and seem to have the best response in PNETs (Strosberg et al., 2011). CAPTEM is administered in a 14-day regimen, with capecitabine taken by mouth twice daily on days 1–14 and temozolomide taken by mouth once daily on days 10–14 on a 28-day cycle that repeats monthly (Ramirez et al., 2016).

Targeted Therapy

Everolimus is a drug that inhibits tumor cell growth, delays progression in metastatic PNETs and gastrointestinal NETs, and has been shown to prolong progression-free survival (Yao et al., 2016). One common side effect of this drug is mouth ulcers (Yao et al., 2016). A rare but potentially fatal adverse reaction is noninfectious pneumonitis. If patients are taking everolimus and present with a cough, immediate investigation with chest x-ray is warranted (Yao et al., 2016). Everolimus has also been shown to delay wound healing and therefore is avoided in the perioperative period (Yao et al., 2016).

Telotristat ethyl is a tryptophan hydroxylase inhibitor used for the treatment of carcinoid syndrome and is the only oral drug approved by the U.S. Food and Drug Administration that has been shown to decrease serotonin levels. Three-times-a-day dosing has shown a significant decrease in diarrhea (Kulke et al., 2017).

Sunitinib has also been shown to slow progression in metastatic low-grade (G1) and intermediate-grade (G2) NETs (Raymond et al., 2011).

Peptide Receptor Radionuclide Therapy

Peptide receptor radionuclide therapy (PRRT) involves systemic administration of radiolabeled SSAs to deliver cytotoxic radioactivity directly to NET cells. The radionuclides ^{68}Ga and ^{111}In used in SSA-based imaging produce beta radiation and do not result in cell damage in low doses (Kwekkeboom et al., 2010). In contrast, the radionuclides lutetium-177 (^{177}Lu) or yttrium-90 (^{90}Y) emit cytotoxic gamma radiation (Kwekkeboom et al., 2010). ^{177}Lu or ^{90}Y can be bound to derivatives of SSA to form substances such as ^{177}Lu-dotatate and ^{90}Y-dotatate, which can be safely administered intravenously to bind to the tumors and cause cell death (Kwekkeboom et al., 2010). This promising new therapy has been shown to extend progression-free survival by approximately three years (Strosberg et al., 2017). PRRT using ^{177}Lu-dotatate is under investigation in several centers in the United States and was approved by the U.S. Food and Drug Administration for treatment of inoperable NETs in early 2018 (Strosberg et al., 2017; U.S. Food and Drug Administration, 2018).

Metaiodobenzylguanidine

Metaiodobenzylguanidine (MIBG) is a compound that can be combined with radioactive iodine-131 (^{131}I) (Campeau et al., 2013). Therapy using ^{131}I-MIBG is effective in controlling growth of NETs in patients who show uptake on iodine-123 (^{123}I)-MIBG scan (Campeau et al., 2013). A ^{123}I-MIBG scan is traditionally used to evaluate NETs of the adrenal glands called pheochromocytomas (Campeau et al., 2013). However, approximately 60% of carcinoid NETs, and to a lesser degree pancreatic islet cell NETs, have positive ^{123}I-MIBG scans and may respond to high-dose ^{131}I-MIBG therapy (Campeau et al., 2013).

Liver-Directed Therapy

Liver-directed therapy is a group of treatment modalities that target metastatic liver disease in patients with NETs. These therapies typically are reserved for patients with unresectable, liver-dominant disease (Woltering et al., 2017). Determination of surgical eligibility and classification of unresectable disease is dependent on the surgeon's experience with NETs. Therefore, patients with extensive disease should be determined to be unresectable only after thorough evaluation by an interprofessional team specializing in NETs (Boudreaux et al., 2014; Woltering et al., 2017).

Ablation Procedures

Hepatic tumors can be destroyed with energy devices by inserting probes and delivering radiofrequency, microwave, or high-voltage direct current, such as with the NanoKnife® (Howe et al., 2017). These therapies can be performed in open surgery, laparoscopically, or percutaneously under x-ray guidance (Howe et al., 2017).

Irreversible electroporation using the NanoKnife causes irreversible damage to tumor cells by creating multiple holes in their cell membrane (Howe et al., 2017). This technique involves insertion of two or more probes into tumors to produce an electrical field using high-voltage direct current. Because the energy source does not create heat in the liver or pancreas, the probes can be used to shrink tumors near delicate structures, such as blood vessels and bile ducts (Howe et al., 2017).

Hepatic Artery Embolization

Hepatic artery embolization refers to multiple liver-directed therapies that use the hepatic artery as an avenue to deliver embolic therapy. The goal of all types of hepatic artery embolization is to occlude the vascular supply to intrahepatic tumors, which derive most of their blood supply from the hepatic artery, not the portal vein (Cives & Strosberg, 2017). Hepatic artery embolization therapies have been shown to be effective in palliation of symptoms resulting from hormonal hypersecretion in patients with liver-dominant metastatic disease (Cives & Strosberg, 2017). Occlusion of blood flow in vessels supplying these tumors results in tumor regression and therefore effectively reduces hormone production (Cives & Strosberg, 2017).

Four types of procedures are commonly used for treatment of liver-dominant metastatic NETs, in each case delivered by angiography. In transarterial embolization, commonly referred to as bland embolization, a clotting agent or microspheres are injected into branches of the hepatic artery that supply the tumor (Kennedy, 2016). Transarterial chemoembolization is identical but adds chemotherapy to the clotting agent or microspheres (Kennedy, 2016). Radioembolization uses microspheres (tiny glass or resin beads) filled with the radioactive isotope ^{90}Y to internally irradiate tumors (Kennedy, 2016). Drug-eluting microsphere beads given transarterially laced with chemotherapy can also be used (Peker, Çiçek, Soydal, Küçük, & Bilgiç, 2015). Studies are ongoing to determine which will be the most effective form of embolotherapy. Additionally, the recommended sequence of these modalities has yet to be identified. Therefore, selection of agents and the sequence of administration are best determined in an interprofessional setting. Known complications include liver abscess due to tumor necrosis or ischemic bile duct strictures, especially in patients who have had multiple procedures (Cives & Strosberg, 2017; Maxwell, O'Dorisio, & Howe, 2016).

The goal of many of these therapies is to control or minimize symptoms caused by hormonal hypersecretion by NETs and minimize disease progression while improving duration and quality of life.

Guidelines for Treatment

Several guidelines for the management and treatment of NETs have been published by national and international organizations. These organizations develop consensus guidelines by forming panels of NET experts and include NCCN, the North American Neuroendocrine Tumor Society, the European Neuroendocrine Tumor Society, and the European Society for Medical Oncology (Anthony et al., 2010; Boudreaux et al., 2010; Howe et al., 2017; Kulke et al., 2010; Öberg, Knigge, Kwekkeboom, & Perren, 2012).

All organizations recommend surgical resection as the primary treatment for most carcinoid tumors of gastrointestinal and bronchopulmonary origins. However, specific recommendations vary by tumor subtype. As advancement in the treatment and management of NETs continues, updated guidelines are continuously released to provide clinicians with the most current recommendations for their patients.

Clinical Trials

Clinical research, including prospective clinical trials as well as retrospective evaluation and analysis of previous outcomes, promotes innovation and development of new therapies to ultimately improve survival in patients with NETs. Although NETs are considered a rare disease, many clinical trials are available and should be considered during treatment planning. All patients should be encouraged to participate in clinical trials and monitor the opening of new trials for which they may be eligible. A comprehensive list is available at the ClinicalTrials.gov website (https://clinicaltrials.gov).

Nursing Care

Symptom Management

Symptom management and control can be challenging in NETs, as many patients present with nonspecific symptoms resembling other diseases, such as irritable bowel syndrome, asthma, Crohn disease, or menopause. Symptoms may result from the overproduction of hormones or other biologically active molecules secreted from NETs or from anatomic mass effects due to tumor bulk (Vinik et al., 2010). Control and reduction of excess hormones produced by NETs are crucial not only to reduce symptoms that affect daily life, but also to reduce the development of life-threatening complications associated with this disease (e.g., carcinoid heart disease). Continuous elevation of hormones produced by NETs, specifically in the case of serotonin, may cause irreversible damage and fibrosis to certain tissues and organs. Thus, every attempt should be made to control symptoms through the control of hormone production. This can be accomplished by decreasing tumor bulk using cytoreductive procedures and use of octreotide or lanreotide to block hormone production (Davar et al., 2017). Telotristat ethyl, a new U.S. Food and Drug Administration–approved medication, can also be used to reduce serotonin levels (Kulke et al., 2017). Surgery and liver-directed therapy have been shown to improve symptoms and survival (Boudreaux et al., 2014). Every attempt should be made to control the release of the hormones, peptides, or amines causing them. Carcinoid syndrome has many triggers, sometimes referred to as the five E's: epinephrine, exercise, ETOH (alcohol), eating, and emotions (Lexicon Pharmaceuticals, Inc., n.d.). Foods with a high content of the vasoactive amines serotonin, tryptamine, dopamine, and norepinephrine should be avoided. These include avocados, bananas, plums, oranges, pineapple, wine, pickled herring, fermented cheese, and salt-dried fish. When educating patients about their diagnosis, it is important to help them identify triggers that can bring on symptoms (Go et al., 2010).

Carcinoid Crisis

Carcinoid crisis is characterized by hypotension, flushing tachycardia, and wheezing and is triggered by many stressors. The stress of medical procedures may cause the release of large amounts of serotonin, producing the combination of symptoms in this potentially life-threatening situation. The treatment of carcinoid crisis is SSAs, fluids, and steroids (Davar et al., 2017). Some institutions choose to administer an octreotide infusion during any invasive procedures, which reduces the risk of carcinoid crisis (Woltering, Wright, et al., 2016).

Nutrition

Nutrition should be a focus when caring for patients with NETs. Excessive amounts of gastrointestinal hormones, peptides, and amines can cause malabsorption, diarrhea, steatorrhea, and altered gastrointestinal motility. SSAs can cause fat malabsorption (steatorrhea) and fat-soluble vitamin (A, D, E, and K) deficiency (Go et al., 2010). The resulting symptoms are weight loss, malnutrition, flushing, abdominal pain, and bloating. A registered dietitian should be part of the interprofessional team, but nurses should be aware of potential problems and familiar with basic interventions. Although some patients can be asymptomatic, others have obvious immediate dietary intervention needs.

For asymptomatic patients, the recommendation is for a healthy diet plan and regular exercise (Go et al., 2010). Symptomatic patients should avoid foods high in amines, spicy foods, and some alcoholic beverages. Foods high in amines include aged cheeses; smoked, salted, or pickled fish or meat; yeast extracts; caffeine; chocolate; sodas; nuts; some pizzas; raspberries; bananas; and avocados. Some of the symptoms can be controlled with SSAs, antidiarrheal medications, or telotristat ethyl. If symptoms persist, patients can keep a diary to identify food triggers. Another nutritional consideration includes the use of pancreatic enzymes to treat the steatorrhea related to the use of SSAs (Go et al., 2010). Monitoring of nutritional status and symptoms in coordination with the healthcare team is essential (Go et al., 2010).

Carcinoid Heart Disease

Carcinoid heart disease is characterized by a combination of symptoms resulting from deposits of plaque-like material on the valves and endocardium of the right side of the heart. Thickening of the leaflets and chordal structures on the affected heart valves occurs. This was first described in the 1950s and affects more than 50% of patients with carcinoid syndrome (Connolly, 2001). These valve changes cause tricuspid and pulmonary valve regurgitation and stenosis. Patients present with right-sided heart failure, which displays symptoms of dyspnea on exertion, fatigue, edema, and ascites. Patients who have carcinoid heart disease have higher serotonin blood levels, which implies that serotonin is a factor in its development (Connolly, 2001).

No recommended guidelines exist for evaluation of carcinoid heart disease. A screening echocardiogram is the current practice in many institutions, with repeated echocardiogram suggested if patients become symptomatic (Connolly, 2001). Diuretics can be useful in the treatment of right-sided heart failure, but with progression, heart valve surgery is an effective treatment and should be considered for symptomatic patients even with metastatic disease. Carcinoid heart disease is not very common but increases the morbidity and mortality for patients who experience it (Connolly, 2001; Davar et al., 2017).

Patient Resources and Advice

It is important to personalize interventions to each patient. Nursing's goal is to help empower patients to take control of their lives. Symptom control; education on diet, exercise, and fatigue; and participation in support groups can all be beneficial at different stages of disease and treatment. Nurses should provide patients with the tools and resources available that address their specific concerns. A thorough patient assessment can indicate how to personalize resources.

Prevention

The etiology of NETs is unknown. Currently, no recommendations for prevention of NETs exist.

Prognosis

Because NETs are typically slow-growing, indolent tumors, excellent long-term survival can be expected with proper management and surveillance. In patients with stage IV, well-differentiated small bowel NETs (i.e., liver metastasis), 5-, 10-, and 20-year survival rates of 87%, 77%, and 41%, respectively, have been reported (Boudreaux et al., 2014). In patients with NETs of all sites who are managed with surgical cytoreduction, 5-, 10-, and 20-year survival rates of 82%, 65%, and 37%, respectively, have been reported (Woltering et al., 2017). The biomarkers pancreastatin and neurokinin A seem to have prognostic significance for survival (Diebold et al., 2012, Woltering, Beyer, et al., 2016).

Surveillance

Surveillance varies widely depending on primary tumor site and stage of disease and from one medical practice to the next. It is thought that the more frequent the surveillance, the more likely a clinician is to diagnose a recurrence or progression. NCCN (2018) guidelines recommend surveillance using routine monitoring of biomarkers and abdominal multiphasic CT or MRI at intervals of 3–12 months.

Survivorship

Survivorship means different things to different people. It is a critical and sometimes the most complex part of the patient journey. It encompasses a mixture of emotions and stressors relating to the continuously varying medical care along the way. The role of the caregiver changes from providing support during diagnosis and treatment to a supportive role with maintenance. This can sometimes be difficult for both parties.

Every survivor has unique challenges. Helping patients identify challenges and providing resources for effective coping will increase chances of success. Resources include support groups, individual counseling, online communities, and friends and family members. Recommending adherence to regular medical checkups and routine surveillance, even if patients feel good, is strongly recommended (Cancer.Net, 2017). The overall goal is to help patients regain independence and be as productive as possible.

Summary

Neuroendocrine tumors are a complex group of rare tumors that range from nonaggressive to aggressive in nature. Patients can present with clinical symptoms due to hormone production or mass effect, or the disease can be silent. Treatment options range from localized to systemic. Surgery often can be lifesaving or life extending. Regardless of the presentation, much is known about these tumors, and an experienced interprofessional team can offer a multitude of therapeutic options. By optimally sequencing these options, clinicians can improve patients' survival and quality of life.

References

Amin, M.B. (Ed.). (2017). *AJCC cancer staging manual* (8th ed.). Chicago, IL: Springer.

Anthony, L.B., Strosberg, J.R., Klimstra, D.S., Maples, W.J., O'Dorisio, T.M., Warner, R.R.P., ... Pommier, R.F. (2010). The NANETS consensus guidelines for the diagnosis and management of gastrointestinal neuroendocrine tumors (NETs): Well-differentiated NETs of the distal colon and rectum. *Pancreas, 39,* 767–774. https://doi.org/10.1097/MPA.0b013e3181ec1261

Boudreaux, J.P. (2011). Surgery for gastroenteropancreatic neuroendocrine tumors (GEPNETS). *Endocrinology and Metabolism Clinics of North America, 40,* 163–171. https://doi.org/10.1016/j.ecl.2010.12.004

Boudreaux, J.P., Klimstra, D.S., Hassan, M.M., Woltering, E.A., Jensen, R.T., Goldsmith, S.J., ... Yao, J.C. (2010). The NANETS consensus guideline for the diagnosis and management of neuroendocrine tumors: Well-differentiated neuroendocrine tumors of the jejunum, ileum, appendix, and cecum. *Pancreas, 39,* 753–766. https://doi.org/10.1097/MPA.0b013e3181ebb2a5

Boudreaux, J.P., Wang, Y.-Z., Diebold, A.E., Frey, D.J., Anthony, L., Uhlhorn, A.P., ... Woltering, E.A. (2014). A single institution's experience with surgical cytoreduction of stage IV, well-differentiated, small bowel neuroendocrine tumors. *Journal of the American College of Surgeons, 218,* 837–844. https://doi.org/10.1016/j.jamcollsurg.2013.12.035

Campeau, R.J., Dowling, A.M., Woltering, E.A., Boudreaux, J.P., Wang, Y.-Z., & Chester, M.M. (2013). Preliminary experience with intra-arterial I-131 MIBG hepatic infusion for progressive metastatic low grade neuroendocrine tumors: An ongoing work-in-progress [Abstract]. *Pancreas, 42,* 371.

Cancer.Net. (2017, August). Neuroendocrine tumor of the pancreas: Survivorship. Retrieved from https://www.cancer.net/cancer-types/neuroendocrine-tumor-pancreas/survivorship

Caplin, M.E., Pavel, M., Ćwikła, J.B., Phan, A.T., Raderer, M., Sedláčková, E., ... Ruszniewski, P. (2014). Lanreotide in metastatic enteropancreatic neuroendocrine tumors. *New England Journal of Medicine, 371,* 224–233. https://doi.org/10.1056/NEJMoa1316158

Chen, C., Yi, X., & He, Y. (2013). Gastro-entero-pancreatic neuroendocrine tumors (GEP-Nets): A review. *Journal of Gastrointestinal and Digestive System, 3,* 154. Retrieved from https://www.omicsonline.org/gastroenteropancreatic-neuroendocrine-tumors-gepnets-a-review-2161-069X-3-154.pdf

Cives, M., & Strosberg, J. (2015). The expanding role of somatostatin analogs in gastroenteropancreatic and lung neuroendocrine tumors. *Drugs, 75,* 847–858. https://doi.org/10.1007/s40265-015-0397-7

Cives, M., & Strosberg, J. (2017). Treatment strategies for metastatic neuroendocrine tumors of the gastrointestinal tract. *Current Treatment Options in Oncology, 18,* 14. https://doi.org/10.1007/s11864-017-0461-5

Connolly, H.M. (2001). Carcinoid heart disease: Medical and surgical considerations. *Cancer Control, 8,* 454–460. https://doi.org/10.1177/107327480100800511

Dasari, A., Shen, C., Halperin, D., Zhao, B., Zhou, S., Xu, Y., ... Yao, J.C. (2017). Trends in the incidence, prevalence, and survival outcomes in patients with neuroendocrine tumors in the United States. *JAMA Oncology, 3,* 1335–1342. https://doi.org/10.1001/jamaoncol.2017.0589

Davar, J., Connolly, H.M., Caplin, M.E., Pavel, M., Zacks, J., Bhattacharyya, S., ... Toumpanakis, C. (2017). Diagnosing and managing carcinoid heart disease in patients with neuroendocrine tumors: An expert statement. *Journal of the American College of Cardiology, 69,* 1288–1304. https://doi.org/10.1016/j.jacc.2016.12.030

Deppen, S.A., Liu, E., Blume, J.D., Clanton, J., Shi, C., Jones-Jackson, L.B., ... Walker, R.C. (2016). Safety and efficacy of ^{68}Ga-DOTATATE PET/CT for diagnosis, staging, and treatment management of neuroendocrine tumors. *Journal of Nuclear Medicine, 57,* 708–714. https://doi.org/10.2967/jnumed.115.163865

Diebold, A.E., Boudreaux, J.P., Wang, Y.-Z., Anthony, L.B., Uhlhorn, A.P., Ryan, P., ... Woltering, E.A. (2012). Neurokinin A levels predict survival in patients with stage IV well differentiated small bowel neuroendocrine neoplasms. *Surgery, 152,* 1172–1176. https://doi.org/10.1016/j.surg.2012.08.057

Díez, M., Teulé, A., & Salazar, R. (2013). Gastroenteropancreatic neuroendocrine tumors: Diagnosis and treatment. *Annals of Gastroenterology, 26,* 29–36. Retrieved from https://www.ncbi.nlm.nih.gov/pmc/articles/PMC3959515

Go, V.L.W., Srihari, P., & Burns, L.A.K. (2010). Nutrition and gastroenteropancreatic neuroendocrine tumors. *Endocrinology and Metabolism Clinics of North America, 39,* 827–837. https://doi.org/10.1016/j.ecl.2010.08.003

Helgadóttir, H., Metz, D.C., Yang, Y.-X., Rhim, A.D., & Björnsson, E.S. (2014). The effects of long-term therapy with proton pump inhibitors on meal stimulated gastrin. *Digestive and Liver Disease, 46,* 125–130. https://doi.org/10.1016/j.dld.2013.09.021

Howe, J.R., Cardona, K., Fraker, D.L., Kebebew, E., Untch, B.R., Wang, Y.-Z., ... Pommier, R.F. (2017). The surgical management of small bowel neuroendocrine tumors: Consensus guidelines of the North American Neuroendocrine Tumor Society. *Pancreas, 46*, 715–731. https://doi.org/10.1097/MPA.0000000000000846

Kennedy, A.S. (2016). Hepatic-directed therapies in patients with neuroendocrine tumors. *Hematology/Oncology Clinics of North America, 30*, 193–207. https://doi.org/10.1016/j.hoc.2015.09.010

Klimstra, D.S., Modlin, I.R., Coppola, D., Lloyd, R.V., & Suster, S. (2010). The pathologic classification of neuroendocrine tumors: A review of nomenclature, grading, and staging systems. *Pancreas, 39*, 707–712. https://doi.org/10.1097/MPA.0b013e3181ec124e

Kulke, M.H., Anthony, L.B., Bushnell, D.L., de Herder, W.W., Goldsmith, S.J., Klimstra, D.S., ... Jensen, R.T. (2010). NANETS treatment guidelines: Well-differentiated neuroendocrine tumors of the stomach and pancreas. *Pancreas, 39*, 735–752. https://doi.org/10.1097/MPA.0b013e3181ebb168

Kulke, M.H., Hörsch, D., Caplin, M.E., Anthony, L.B., Bergsland, E., Öberg, K., ... Pavel, M. (2017). Telotristat ethyl, a tryptophan hydroxylase inhibitor for the treatment of carcinoid syndrome. *Journal of Clinical Oncology, 35*, 14–23. https://doi.org/10.1200/JCO.2016.69.2780

Kunz, P.L., Reidy-Lagunes, D., Anthony, L.B., Bertino, E.M., Brendtro, K., Chan, J.A., ... Yao, J.C. (2013). Consensus guidelines for the management and treatment of neuroendocrine tumors. *Pancreas, 42*, 557–577. https://doi.org/10.1097/MPA.0b013e31828e34a4

Kwekkeboom, D.J., Kam, B.L., van Essen, M., Teunissen, J.J.M., van Eijck, C.H.J., Valkema, R., ... Krenning, E.P. (2010). Somatostatin receptor-based imaging and therapy of gastroenteropancreatic neuroendocrine tumors. *Endocrine-Related Cancer, 17*, R53–R73. https://doi.org/10.1677/ERC-09-0078

Lexicon Pharmaceuticals, Inc. (n.d.). Carcinoid syndrome symptoms. Retrieved from https://www.aboutcarcinoid.com/carcinoid-syndrome-symptoms

Maxwell, J.E., & Howe, J.R. (2015). Imaging in neuroendocrine tumors: An update for the clinician. *International Journal of Endocrine Oncology, 2*, 159–168. https://doi.org/10.2217/ije.14.40

Maxwell, J.E., O'Dorisio, T.M., & Howe, J.R. (2016). Biochemical diagnosis and preoperative imaging of gastroenteropancreatic neuroendocrine tumors. *Surgical Oncology Clinics of North America, 25*, 171–194. https://doi.org/10.1016/j.soc.2015.08.008

Maxwell, J.E., Sherman, S.K., O'Dorisio, T.M., Bellizzi, A.M., & Howe, J.R. (2016). Liver-directed surgery of neuroendocrine metastases: What is the optimal strategy? *Surgery, 159*, 320–335. https://doi.org/10.1016/j.surg.2015.05.040

Modlin, I.M., Kidd, M., Latich, I., Zikusoka, M.N., & Shapiro, M.D. (2005). Current status of gastrointestinal carcinoids. *Gastroenterology, 128*, 1717–1751. https://doi.org/10.1053/j.gastro.2005.03.038

Modlin, I.M., Oberg, K., Chung, D.C., Jensen, R.T., de Herder, W.W., Thakker, R.V., ... Sundin, A. (2008). Gastroenteropancreatic neuroendocrine tumours. *Lancet Oncology, 9*, 61–72. https://doi.org/10.1016/S1470-2045(07)70410-2

National Comprehensive Cancer Network. (2018). *NCCN Clinical Practice Guidelines in Oncology (NCCN Guidelines®): Neuroendocrine and adrenal tumors* [v.2.2018]. Retrieved from https://www.nccn.org/professionals/physician_gls/pdf/neuroendocrine.pdf

Öberg, K., Knigge, U., Kwekkeboom, D., & Perren, A. (2012). Neuroendocrine gastro-entero-pancreatic tumors: ESMO clinical practice guidelines for diagnosis, treatment and follow-up. *Annals of Oncology, 23*(Suppl. 7), vii124–vii130. https://doi.org/10.1093/annonc/mds295

Peker, A., Çiçek, O., Soydal, Ç., Küçük, N.Ö., & Bilgiç, S. (2015). Radioembolization with yttrium-90 resin microspheres for neuroendocrine tumor liver metastases. *Diagnostic and Interventional Radiology, 21*, 54–59. https://doi.org/10.5152/dir.2014.14036

Raines, D., Chester, M., Diebold, A.E., Mamikunian, P., Anthony, C.T., Mamikunian, G., & Woltering, E.A. (2012). A prospective evaluation of the effect of chronic proton pump inhibitor use on plasma biomarker levels in humans. *Pancreas, 41,* 508–511. https://doi.org/10.1097/MPA.0b013e318243a0b6

Ramage, J.K., Ahmed, A., Ardill, J., Bax, N., Breen, D.J., Caplin, M.E., ... Grossman, A.B. (2012). Guidelines for the management of gastroenteropancreatic neuroendocrine (including carcinoid) tumours (NETs). *Gut, 61,* 6–32. https://doi.org/10.1136/gutjnl-2011-300831

Ramirez, R.A., Beyer, D.T., Chauhan, A., Boudreaux, J.P., Wang, Y.-Z., & Woltering, E.A. (2016). The role of capecitabine/temozolomide in metastatic neuroendocrine tumors. *Oncologist, 21,* 671–675. https://doi.org/10.1634/theoncologist.2015-0470

Raymond, E., Dahan, L., Raoul, J.-L., Bang, Y.-J., Borbath, I., Lombard-Bohas, C., ... Ruszniewski, P. (2011). Sunitinib malate for the treatment of pancreatic neuroendocrine tumors. *New England Journal of Medicine, 364,* 501–513. https://doi.org/10.1056/NEJMoa1003825

Rindi, G., Arnold, R., Bosman, F.T., Capella, C., Klimstra, D.S., Klöppel, G., ... Solcia, E. (2010). Nomenclature and classification of neuroendocrine neoplasms of the digestive system. In F.T. Bosman, F. Carneiro, R. Hruban, & N.D. Theise (Eds.), *WHO classification of tumours of the digestive system* (4th ed., pp. 13–145). Lyon, France: IARC Press.

Rinke, A., Müller, H.-H., Schade-Brittinger, C., Klose, K.-J., Barth, P., Wied, M., ... Arnold, R. (2009). Placebo-controlled, double-blind, prospective, randomized study on the effect of octreotide LAR in the control of tumor growth in patients with metastatic neuroendocrine midgut tumors: A report from the PROMID Study Group. *Journal of Clinical Oncology, 27,* 4656–4663. https://doi.org/10.1200/JCO.2009.22.8510

Saif, M.W., Larson, H., Kaley, K., & Shaib, W. (2010). Chronic octreotide therapy can induce pancreatic insufficiency: A common but under-recognized adverse effect. *Expert Opinion on Drug Safety, 9,* 867–873. https://doi.org/10.1517/14740338.2010.510130

Singh, S., Sivajohanathan, D., Asmis, T., Cho, C., Hammad, N., Law, C., ... Zbuk, K. (2017). Systemic therapy in incurable gastroenteropancreatic neuroendocrine tumours: A clinical practice guideline. *Current Oncology, 24,* 249. https://doi.org/10.3747/co.24.3634

Strosberg, J., El-Haddad, G., Wolin, E., Hendifar, A., Yao, J., Chasen, B., ... Krenning, E. (2017). Phase 3 trial of ^{177}Lu-dotatate for midgut neuroendocrine tumors. *New England Journal of Medicine, 376,* 125–135. https://doi.org/10.1056/NEJMoa1607427

Strosberg, J.R., Fine, R.L., Choi, J., Nasir, A., Coppola, D., Chen, D.-T., ... Kvols, L. (2011). First-line chemotherapy with capecitabine and temozolomide in patients with metastatic pancreatic endocrine carcinomas. *Cancer, 117,* 268–275. https://doi.org/10.1002/cncr.25425

Turaga, K.K., & Kvols, L.K. (2011). Recent progress in the understanding, diagnosis, and treatment of gastroenteropancreatic neuroendocrine tumors. *CA: A Cancer Journal for Clinicians, 61,* 113–132. https://doi.org/10.3322/caac.20097

U.S. Food and Drug Administration. (2018, January 26). FDA approves lutetium Lu 177 dotatate for treatment of GEP-NETS. Retrieved from https://www.fda.gov/drugs/informationondrugs/approveddrugs/ucm594105.htm

Vinik, A.I., & Chaya, C. (2016). Clinical presentation and diagnosis of neuroendocrine tumors. *Hematology/Oncology Clinics of North America, 30,* 21–48. https://doi.org/10.1016/j.hoc.2015.08.006

Vinik, A.I., Woltering, E.A., Warner, R.R.P., Caplin, M., O'Dorisio, T.M., Wiseman, G.A., ... Go, V.L.W. (2010). NANETS consensus guidelines for the diagnosis of neuroendocrine tumor. *Pancreas, 39,* 713–734. https://doi.org/10.1097/MPA.0b013e3181ebaffd

Woltering, E.A., Beyer, D.T., Thiagarajan, R., Ramirez, R.A., Wang, Y.-Z., Ricks, M.J., & Boudreaux, J.P. (2016). Elevated plasma pancreastatin, but not chromogranin A, predicts survival in neuroendocrine tumors of the duodenum. *Journal of the American College of Surgeons, 222,* 534–542. https://doi.org/10.1016/j.jamcollsurg.2015.12.014

Woltering, E.A., Vinik, A.I., O'Dorisio, T.M., Go, V.L.W., & Mamikunian, G. (2012). *Neuroendocrine tumors: A comprehensive guide to diagnosis and management* (5th ed.). Inglewood, CA: Inter Science Institute.

Woltering, E.A., Voros, B.A., Beyer, D.T., Wang, Y.-Z., Thiagarajan, R., Ryan, P., ... Boudreaux, J.P. (2017). Aggressive surgical approach to the management of neuroendocrine tumors: A report of 1,000 surgical cytoreductions by a single institution. *Journal of the American College of Surgeons, 224,* 434–447. https://doi.org/10.1016/j.jamcollsurg.2016.12.032

Woltering, E.A., Wright, A.E., Stevens, M.A., Wang, Y.-Z., Boudreaux, J.P., Mamikunian, G., ... Kaye, A.D. (2016). Development of effective prophylaxis against intraoperative carcinoid crisis. *Journal of Clinical Anesthesia, 32,* 189–193. https://doi.org/10.1016/j.jclinane.2016.03.008

Yao, J.C., Fazio, N., Singh, S., Buzzoni, R., Carnaghi, C., Wolin, E., ... Pavel, M.E. (2016). Everolimus for the treatment of advanced, non-functional neuroendocrine tumours of the lung or gastrointestinal tract (RADIANT-4): A randomised, placebo-controlled, phase 3 study. *Lancet, 387,* 968–977. https://doi.org/10.1016/S0140-6736(15)00817-X

Yao, J.C., Hassan, M., Phan, A., Dagohoy, C., Leary, C., Mares, J.E., ... Evans, D.B. (2008). One hundred years after "carcinoid": Epidemiology of and prognostic factors for neuroendocrine tumors in 35,825 cases in the United States. *Journal of Clinical Oncology, 26,* 3063–3072. https://doi.org/10.1200/JCO.2007.15.4377

CHAPTER 6

Primary Liver and Biliary Tract Cancers

Jessica MacIntyre, ARNP, NP-C, AOCNP®

Introduction

The liver is the largest internal organ, lying under the right ribs just beneath the right lung. It is divided into the right and left lobes. Only cancers that start in the liver are called liver cancer (also termed *primary liver cancer*) (American Cancer Society [ACS], n.d.). Liver cancer includes two major types: hepatocellular carcinoma (HCC) and intrahepatic bile duct cancer (National Cancer Institute [NCI], 2018a). Other primary cancers that metastasize to the liver are not considered primary liver cancer. Figure 6-1 illustrates the anatomy of the biliary tract.

Biliary tract cancers are rare but heterogeneous and comprise intrahepatic cholangiocarcinoma, extrahepatic cholangiocarcinoma, and gallbladder cancer (Ahn & Bekaii-Saab, 2017). Gallbladder cancer is a disease in which malignant (cancer) cells form in the tissues of the gallbladder (NCI, 2018c). Intrahepatic bile duct cancer, or intrahepatic cholangiocarcinoma, forms in the bile ducts inside the liver, and extrahepatic cholangiocarcinoma consists of cancers in the hilum region of the liver and distal bile duct region. Perihilar bile duct cancer develops where the right and left bile ducts exit the liver and join to form the common hepatic duct, while distal cholangiocarcinoma occurs in the common bile duct, which passes through the pancreas and ends in the small intestine (NCI, 2018b). Hilar bile duct cancers are also called Klatskin tumors. Biliary tract cancers are invasive adenocarcinomas that arise from the epithelial lining of the gallbladder and the intra- and extrahepatic bile ducts (Rakić et al., 2014). The gallbladder and ampulla of Vater are considered structures of the biliary tract system, and hence, malignancies of those parts usually are included in research and publications involving cholangiocarcinoma (Recio-Boiles & Babiker, 2018). However, ampullary cancers are beyond the scope of this chapter.

Figure 6-1. Anatomy of the Biliary Tract

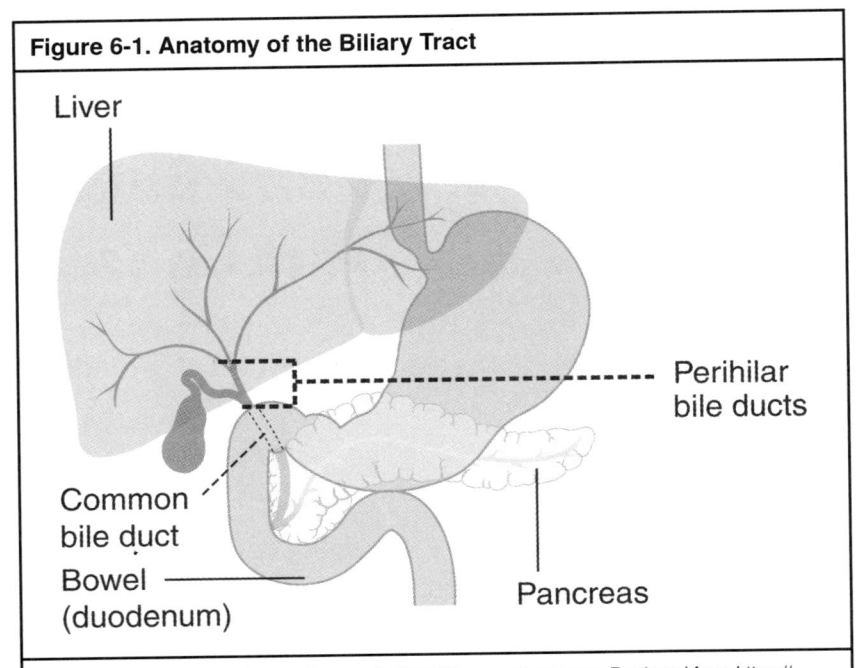

Note. Image courtesy of Cancer Research UK/Wikimedia Commons. Retrieved from https://commons.wikimedia.org/wiki/File:Diagram_showing_the_position_of_the_perihilar_bile_ducts_CRUK_357.svg. Used under the Creative Commons Attribution-ShareAlike 4.0 International (CC BY-SA 4.0) license (https://creativecommons.org/licenses/by-sa/4.0/legalcode).

Primary Liver Cancer

Incidence and Epidemiology

Incidence and mortality rates for cancer overall are declining, but rates for HCC are increasing (Ryerson et al., 2016). Incidence rates have tripled since 1980 and are three times higher in men than in women (ACS, 2018a). In the United States, 42,220 new cases of liver cancer (including intrahepatic bile duct cancers) were estimated for 2018, approximately three-fourths of which will be HCC. The estimated deaths for liver cancer in 2018 were 30,200 (ACS, 2018b). Liver cancer is a leading cause of cancer deaths worldwide, accounting for more than 600,000 deaths each year, and is more common in sub-Saharan Africa and Southeast Asia than in the United States (ACS, 2018b).

Etiology and Risk Factors

HCC carcinogenesis is a complex process that can involve various modifications to a number of molecular pathways as well as genetic alterations, ultimately leading to malignant transformation and HCC disease progression (Sanyal, Yoon, & Lencioni, 2010). Multiple factors are responsible for the initiation and progression of HCC, including virus-induced, alcohol-induced, and fungi-induced hepatocarcinogenesis; obesity; and type 2 diabetes (Dutta & Mahato, 2017).

The most important risk factors for liver cancer in the United States are chronic infection with hepatitis B virus (HBV) or hepatitis C virus (HCV), heavy alcohol consumption, obesity, diabetes, and tobacco smoking (ACS, 2016). Patients with chronic liver disease are at the highest risk for developing HCC (Wang et al., 2015). Chronic HBV infection is the leading cause of HCC in Asia and Africa, whereas HCV infection is the leading cause in Europe, Japan, and North America (National Comprehensive Cancer Network® [NCCN®], 2018). Some nonviral causes include hereditary hemochromatosis, porphyria cutanea tarda, alpha-1 antitrypsin deficiency, Wilson disease, and stage IV biliary cirrhosis (Benson et al., 2017). Additionally, contamination of foodstuffs with aflatoxin B_1 can cause liver cirrhosis and has been reported in 50% of HCC tumors in southern Africa, where aflatoxin B_1 is a known risk factor for developing HCC (Sanyal et al., 2010).

Signs and Symptoms

Because most patients with HCC have chronic viral infections, routine imaging is performed for early detection. Typically, these patients are followed by their hepatologist and undergo routine liver ultrasounds and blood tests. Patients may be asymptomatic at the time of diagnosis and tend to report vague symptoms such as fatigue or malaise, which may be more related to the virus (HBV or HCV) than the malignancy. Other symptoms patients may present with, especially in advanced disease, include abdominal pain, increased abdominal girth, jaundice, fever, and weight loss. Enlargement of the liver is the most common physical sign (ACS, 2018a), and ascites can also be present.

Diagnostic Evaluation

Because of viral infections such as HBV and HCV causing increasing risk of HCC, NCCN (2018) recommends screening with ultrasound and optional alpha–fetoprotein (AFP) testing every six months. Some disagreement exists between experts on the use of AFP as a screening tool for high-risk individuals (patients with cirrhosis due to HBV, alcohol, genetic hemochromatosis, primary biliary cirrhosis, alpha-1 antitrypsin deficiency, and other causes). Ultrasound is generally used worldwide, mostly because of its ease of approach, lack of radiation, and relatively inexpensive cost compared to computed tomography (CT) and magnetic resonance imaging (MRI) (Wang et al., 2015). Additional imaging (abdominal multiphasic CT or MRI) is recommended in the setting of a rising AFP or following identification of a liver mass nodule 10 mm or greater on ultrasound. These recommendations are based on multiple guidelines from the American Association for the Study of Liver Diseases, the Organ Procurement and Transplantation Network, and the Liver Imaging Reporting and Data System (Marrero et al., 2018).

HCC lesions are characterized by arterial hypervascularity and derive their blood supply mainly from the hepatic artery (NCCN, 2018). Using a multiphasic abdominal contrast-enhanced CT or MRI (including arterial and portal venous phase) can provide the perfusion characteristics, extent and number of lesions, vascular anatomy, and presence of extrahepatic disease. This will also help differentiate between HCC and metastatic liver disease from another primary tumor.

According to NCCN (2018), if multiphasic contrast-enhanced imaging does not detect a mass or if the observation is definitely benign, the patient should return to a screening program (e.g., ultrasound and AFP in six months). If the diagnostic imaging test is suspicious for a false positive, then a different imaging method with or without AFP may be considered. However, if the observation is inconclusive (i.e., not definitely HCC but not definitely benign), then interprofessional discussion and individualized workup may be undertaken, including additional imaging or biopsy (NCCN, 2018).

Fluorodeoxyglucose positron-emission tomography (PET) is a functional imaging tool that provides metabolic information. PET-CT is not recommended for detection of HCC because of limited sensitivity; however, it may assist with prognosis. A meta-analysis of 22 studies with 1,721 patients with HCC showed usefulness of PET-CT for predicting prognosis (i.e., overall survival [OS] and disease-free survival) but low sensitivity for detecting HCC (Sun et al., 2016). Therefore, NCCN (2018) does not recommend PET-CT for detection of HCC. For CT- or MRI-detected HCC that has increased metabolic activity on PET-CT, higher intralesional standardized uptake value is a marker of biologic aggressiveness and may predict poorer response to locoregional therapies (NCCN, 2018).

In addition to imaging workup, blood tests performed include a complete blood count, complete metabolic panel with liver profile, and coagulation studies. If bilirubin or liver function is elevated, coagulation may be affected, and attention should be given to these laboratory results because invasive or surgical procedures may be recommended. Other laboratory work to be considered to complete the workup includes a hepatitis panel for detection of HBV or HCV, if not already known. If the patient tests positive for HBV or HCV, a viral load and HCV antibodies, respectively, should be performed for consideration of antiviral therapy.

The tumor marker related to HCC, as mentioned earlier, is AFP. As a frontline HCC screening tool, AFP is the most frequently used tumor marker worldwide. However, not all HCCs have an elevated AFP. AFP is found elevated in the blood of 50%–70% of people who have HCC (Cancer.Net, 2017). Conditions that can falsely elevate AFP are chronic liver disease without HCC and other malignant tumors. Other tumor markers that can assist in those without elevation in AFP are AFP-L3 fraction and descarboxyprothrombin, also known as protein induced by vitamin K absence or antagonist II (known as PIVKA-II). Increased concentrations of these markers are associated with features of poor prognosis, including large tumors, invasion of the portal vein, and poor differentiation of HCC cells (Bruix, Reig, & Sherman, 2016).

Differentiating between intrahepatic cholangiocarcinoma and HCC can be difficult. Testing AFP levels can be considered, especially if the patient has chronic liver disease. A number of mixed HCC and intrahepatic cholangiocarcinomas may also present with elevated AFP (NCCN, 2018).

Obtaining the diagnosis of HCC via biopsy may not be required. NCCN (2018) provides recommendations for when to biopsy a patient with a potential HCC diagnosis: the lesion is suspicious for malignancy on imaging but characteristics are not that of HCC, or the lesion meets imaging criteria but the patient is not at high risk for HCC or has conditions associated with formation of nonmalignant nodules that may be confused with HCC during imaging. Otherwise, if imaging correlates with characteristics of HCC and AFP is elevated, a biopsy is not needed.

Histology

HCC accounts for 90% of primary liver cancer cases (NCI, 2018a). One subtype of HCC is fibrolamellar, which occurs more often in women and has a better clinical course than HCC. Other histologic classifications of primary liver cancer include intrahepatic cholangiocarcinoma, angiosarcoma and hemangiosarcoma, hepatoblastoma (occurs more often in children than in adults), mixed hepatocellular cholangiocarcinoma, and undifferentiated (NCI, 2018a).

Clinical Staging

Three types of staging systems are used to classify HCC: the Barcelona Clinic Liver Cancer (BCLC) staging system, the Okuda staging system, and the American Joint Committee on Cancer (AJCC) staging system. The Okuda staging system mostly serves to recognize end-stage disease.

The BCLC staging system is the most accepted staging system for HCC and is useful in the staging of early tumors (Holzwanger & Madoff, 2018). It is endorsed in the American Association for the Study of Liver Diseases guidelines (Marrero et al., 2018). The variables included are tumor stage, functional status of the liver, physical status,

and cancer-related symptoms. It also incorporates the Okuda stage and Child-Pugh score (Subramaniam, Kelley, & Venook, 2013). The stages are as follows:
- Stage 0 (very early stage)—asymptomatic early tumors in which surgical resection is offered
- Stage A (early stage)—asymptomatic early tumors in which surgical resection, ablation, or transplantation is offered
- Stage B (intermediate stage)—asymptomatic multinodular tumors in which arterial therapies are offered
- Stage C (advanced stage)—symptomatic or invasive tumors in which systemic or palliative therapies are offered
- Stage D (end-stage disease)—symptomatic tumors in which supportive care is offered

The AJCC staging system includes the tumor-node-metastasis (TNM) classifications for staging, but its limitation is that is does not include liver function and, as a result, is not widely used for liver cancer. TNM staging may be useful in prognostic prediction after liver resection.

AJCC prognostic staging groups for liver cancer are as follows (Abou-Alfa, Pawlik, Shindoh, & Vauthey, 2017):
- Stage IA: T1a N0 M0
- Stage IB: T1b N0 M0
- Stage II: T2 N0 M0
- Stage IIIA: T3 N0 M0
- Stage IIIB: T4 N0 M0
- Stage IVA: Any T, N1 M0
- Stage IVB: Any T, Any N, M1

Treatment
Surgery and Minimally Invasive Procedures

Standard treatment options for adult patients with BCLC stage 0, A, and B primary liver cancer include surgical resection, liver transplantation, and ablation. As mentioned, many variables factor into which treatment option is recommended, such as characteristics of the liver and tumor. The Child-Pugh score offers an estimate of liver function; however, it has been suggested to be more useful as a tool to rule out liver resection (i.e., for identifying patients with substantially decompensated liver disease) (NCCN, 2018). The Child-Pugh score includes the clinical and laboratory criteria of encephalopathy, ascites, bilirubin, albumin, and prothrombin time. It classifies patients as having compensated liver disease (class A) or decompensated liver disease (classes B or C). The following are the classes of Child-Pugh scores when calculated (Bruix et al., 2016):
- Class A = 5–6 points (least severe liver disease)
- Class B = 7–9 points (moderately severe liver disease)
- Class C = 10–15 points (most severe liver disease)

The Model for End-Stage Liver Disease (MELD) is another system for evaluation of hepatic reserve. MELD accounts for serum bilirubin, creatinine, and international normalized ratio. It is used by the United Network for Organ Sharing and helps to determine the need for transplant for patients on the liver transplant waiting list by estimating their risk of death within three months (Bruix et al., 2016). Additionally, assessments of patient performance status also must be considered. Comorbidity is an independent predictor of perioperative mortality (NCCN, 2018). For this reason, it is important to discuss the treatment plan for these patients in an interprofessional tumor conference with all team members present. This includes but is not limited to representatives from radiology, pathology, hepatology, gastroenterology, interventional radiology, transplant surgery, surgical oncology, and medical oncology.

Surgery is no longer the only first-line treatment. Resection, transplantation, and ablation provide excellent results for single lesions 2 cm or smaller (T1a stage) in patients with preserved liver function (Bruix et al., 2016). There is no straightforward approach to managing and treating patients with HCC. Treatment tends to be individualized for each patient. Although liver transplantation is an excellent treatment for HCC, the number of patients waiting for a liver exceeds the number of available grafts (Sapisochin & Bruix, 2017). As a result, other treatment approaches are offered during the transplant-waiting period, commonly referred to as *bridge therapies*, and will be discussed later in this chapter.

Partial hepatectomy (surgery to remove part of the liver) is a potentially curative therapy for patients with a solitary tumor of any size with no evidence of gross vascular invasion (NCCN, 2018). The presence of extrahepatic metastasis is considered to be a contraindication for resection. Common sites of metastases include the lungs, abdominal lymph nodes, peritoneum, and bone (NCCN, 2018). Adequate liver reserve is also an important criterion to consider for patients undergoing hepatic resection, especially in patients with underlying cirrhosis.

For patients with a low MELD score (awaiting transplantation) and growing and changing liver tumors via imaging with correlated increasing AFP, a locoregional approach can be considered and is referred to as bridge therapy. Bridge therapy is used to decrease tumor progression and the transplant waiting list dropout rate (NCCN, 2018). Patients who do not meet liver transplant criteria can also be downstaged with locoregional therapies (NCCN, 2018).

Transarterial chemotherapy and radiofrequency ablation (RFA) are other options to consider. They are classified as locoregional therapies because they are targeted to specific areas rather than a systemic therapy approach. Locoregional therapies are the preferred treatment approach for patients who are not amenable to surgery or liver transplantation (NCCN, 2018).

RFA consists of inserting a needle either percutaneously, laparoscopically, or through an open approach and applying either heat (RFA) or microwave energy, also called *microwave ablation*. Another modality often discussed is cryoablation (using cold), but it is not typically used in the liver (Holzwanger & Madoff, 2018).

Ablation procedures are guided via CT or ultrasound to locate the tumor and treat that exact area. A thin probe or needle that emits heat (RFA) or microwave energy (microwave ablation) is inserted into the tumor, and a margin of normal tissue is also treated. The probe introduces heat or microwave energy that ablates (destroys) the tumor (NCI, 2018a).

Arterial therapies can be performed using doxorubicin drug-eluting beads, radioactive beads, yttrium-90 (^{90}Y), or bland embolization (cutting off blood supply by using an embolic particle that causes ischemia). The procedure consists of inserting a catheter via the femoral artery (groin) or radial artery (arm) and using fluoroscopy guidance to thread the catheter to the area in the liver that requires treatment. Then, the treatment is inserted directly into the tumor. Some contraindications for arterial therapies include high bilirubin levels (greater than 2 or 3 mg/dl, depending on the procedure), portal venous thrombosis, Child-Pugh C liver function, and extrahepatic disease (NCCN, 2018).

NCCN (2018) recommends ablation be considered for patients with tumors 3 cm or smaller (if location is accessible). For patients with 3–5 cm lesions, a combination of ablation (if location is accessible) and other locoregional therapies is considered. Patients with unresectable or inoperable lesions greater than 5 cm should be considered for treatment using arterially directed therapies or systemic therapies.

Preoperative management: During the preoperative period, patients may be recommended to undergo additional workup to ensure readiness for surgery. The workup is even more extensive for patients undergoing a liver transplantation; a liver transplant coordinator usually handles the coordination and care of these patients. For patients undergoing liver resection or a locoregional therapy, laboratory work, anesthesia clearance (including cardiology and respiratory examinations), and evaluation or bridging of coagulation problems should be addressed. Patients should receive education on the type of procedure/surgery, typical length of time of the procedure/surgery, length of stay at the hospital, and possible postoperative complications. The possibility also exists that the procedure/surgery will be aborted intraoperatively if the tumor is found to be inaccessible or unresectable. Ensuring awareness of this prior to treatment will provide patients the understanding that the procedure/surgery may not be definitive despite the staging workup and extensive preparation.

The preoperative time is a time of anxiety for patients (especially for patients on the liver transplant waiting list) because there will be a period of waiting after the first visit until the time of the surgery. Reassuring patients and providing continuous communication that precautions are being taken to ultimately improve their safety and outcomes during the procedure/surgery will offer some relief to patients and their caregivers (Sadati et al., 2013).

Postoperative management: Postsurgical outcomes appear to improve in patients treated in high-specialty centers, with a 75% rate of extended hepatic resection and 80% rate of R0 resections (Squadroni et al., 2017). Variable postoperative complications can be seen depending on the type of surgery performed. Thromboembolic disease risk is high in patients with gastrointestinal cancer because of a hypercoagulable state. Prophylactic low-molecular-weight heparin is recommended following surgery, depending on the patient's history, to prevent a postsurgical embolism. Nurses, however, should be knowledgeable of underlying liver disease and increased bleeding risk with anticoagulant use.

Liver failure is also a risk during the postoperative period, depending on the extent of liver resection, and especially after transplant. This is a critical time with frequent monitoring of liver function tests, and unusual increases in values should be reported immediately. Other signs that should be noted to prevent worsening of postsurgical complications are painless jaundice, amber-colored urine, and clay-colored stools.

Depending on the output results, drains may be removed or kept in place if biliary leak is a concern. Educating patients on the care and maintenance of drainage systems by recording outputs and color will help providers determine the timing of drain removal.

Intake and output will also need to be monitored by nurses and patients during the postoperative period to prevent electrolyte imbalances, nutritional complications, and dehydration. Some patients may require a nasogastric tube to allow for stomach decompression and may be supported with total parenteral nutrition including lipids to support them during the initial days to weeks postoperatively.

Increasing physical activity will assist in preventing embolism and hospital-acquired pneumonia. Additionally, monitoring for possible infections is also critical to the recovery of patients who have undergone an invasive procedure or surgical operation. Patients with comorbidities such as diabetes and older age are at increased risk. Incision sites should be monitored frequently for erythema, edema, and drainage.

Pain control is also an important aspect in the surgical or procedural postoperative setting. A patient-controlled analgesia pump may be ordered to allow for optimal pain control management by the patient and provider. Frequent assessment of pain levels will assist nurses in reporting changes to providers early on to improve discharge outcomes.

Communication regarding postdischarge care is one of the most important and overlooked areas in the postoperative care of these patients. Depending on the intraoperative findings and preliminary pathology, coordination of postsurgical care at home will be critical to continuation of the patient's recovery and consideration of treatment with other modalities, such as systemic therapies and immunosuppressants. It is essential to ensure that a postsurgical follow-up appointment has been secured prior to discharge to avoid delays in treatment and readmission to the hospital. In addition, ensuring social support at home is critical, especially for liver transplant recipients (Kapritsou et al., 2014).

Chemotherapy

Minimal advances have occurred in the treatment of HCC. However, systemic therapy has often been recommended only for those with very advanced disease (NCCN, 2018). Clinical studies evaluating the use of cytotoxic chemotherapy in the treatment of patients with advanced HCC have typically reported low response rates, and evidence for a favorable impact of chemotherapy on OS is lacking (NCCN, 2018). One of the agents approved in the advanced setting is sorafenib, an oral multikinase inhibitor. It was approved based on the SHARP trial (Llovet et al., 2008), which enrolled 602 patients with advanced HCC and randomized them to either sorafenib or best supportive care. Results showed that median OS was significantly longer in the sorafenib arm than the placebo arm (10.7 months vs. 7.9 months). The most common adverse events associated with sorafenib include diarrhea, weight loss, and hand-foot syndrome. NCCN (2018) recommends sorafenib as a first-line treatment for patients with advanced HCC and Child-Pugh A liver function.

For second-line treatment, NCCN (2018) recommends regorafenib (an oral multikinase inhibitor) as a category 1 option based on the international phase 3 RESORCE trial (Bruix et al., 2017). The trial assessed efficacy and safety in 573 patients with HCC and Child-Pugh A liver function who progressed on sorafenib. Median survival results showed 10.6 months with regorafenib versus 7.8 months in the placebo arm. Use of regorafenib also resulted in improved OS, progression-free survival, time to progression, objective response, and disease control. The most common adverse events seen were hypertension, hand-foot syndrome, fatigue, and diarrhea.

Another treatment that can be considered in the advanced setting that has shown modest results is the FOLFOX4 regimen. This regimen includes the use of infusional 5-fluorouracil, leucovorin, and oxaliplatin. In a trial by Qin et al. (2013), the endpoint of OS was not met, but progression-free survival was greater in the FOLFOX4 arm versus the doxorubicin arm (NCCN, 2018). Because of the lack of approved regimens and small benefits seen in survival from the standard-of-care treatments, a clinical trial should always be recommended in this patient population when available (Ahn & Bekaii-Saab, 2017).

The oncology nursing role in this setting lies in assessment of oral treatment adherence and side effects, management of symptoms, and advocacy for palliative care when recommended. In reference to side effects with the aforementioned regimens, diarrhea, fatigue, and hand-foot syndrome are most common. Additionally, educating patients and their caregivers on adherence to oral treatments will assist in optimizing their response to treatment and, hence, quality of life. Early introduction of supportive and palliative care measures should also be considered to assist patients in continuing treatment and improving quality of life.

Radiation Therapy

Advances in external beam radiation therapy (EBRT), such as intensity-modulated radiation therapy, have allowed for enhanced delivery of higher radiation doses to the tumor while sparing surrounding critical tissue. Stereotactic body radiation therapy (SBRT) is an advanced EBRT technique that delivers large ablative doses of radiation (NCCN, 2018). Growing evidence (primarily from nonrandomized controlled trials) is supporting the usefulness of SBRT for patients with unresectable, locally advanced, or recurrent HCC (NCCN, 2018). NCCN (2018) recommends consideration of SBRT as an alternative to ablation or embolization techniques when these therapies have failed or are contraindicated in patients with unresectable disease characterized as extensive or otherwise unsuitable for liver transplantation or those with local disease who are not candidates for surgery because of performance status or comorbidity. Radiation therapy also has a role in the palliative setting for patients with HCC who have metastatic disease to the bone or brain (NCCN, 2018).

Transarterial radioembolization or selective internal radiation therapy with ^{90}Y was discussed earlier as a locoregional treatment. ^{90}Y is a beta emitter with a half-life of 64.2 hours (Holzwanger & Madoff, 2018). In radioembolization, tiny glass or resin beads called microspheres are placed inside the blood vessels that feed a tumor in order to block the supply of blood to cancer cells. Once these ^{90}Y microspheres become lodged at the tumor site, they deliver a high dose of radiation that is limited to the tumor and not to normal tissues. In this procedure, the radiation oncologist determines and prepares the dose, and the interventional radiologist performs the pre-^{90}Y mapping procedure and intraoperative ^{90}Y delivery procedure, with the assistance of the radiation oncologist. Some radiation safety considerations exist when treating patients undergoing transarterial radioembolization. For one week after the procedure, patients should limit contact with others. They should not sleep in the same bed, use public transportation that requires them to sit next to another person for more than two hours, or come in close contact with children or pregnant women. Patients are also at risk for ulcers due to bead dislodgment and are placed on antacids for prevention. In addition, patients should be provided opioids prior to discharge because the procedure can produce pain, and they should also be informed of the late onset of fatigue that can be seen after the procedure.

Nursing care for patients undergoing EBRT includes education about the timing of radiation and the different phases of preparation (i.e., planning and simulation) prior to starting treatment, as the time leading up to treatment may be delayed. Oncology nurses should also be advocates for patients before, during, and after treatment because patients will see many providers and can become lost to follow-up care. It is important to maintain timing of procedures so that patients can plan accordingly and decrease delays in treatment. Communication among the radiation oncologist, interventional radiologist, and medical oncologist should also remain open so that if side effects arise, supportive care can be provided (Sur & Sharma, 2017).

Immunotherapy

Immunotherapy is making an impact in many cancers, including HCC. Nivolumab, a programmed cell death protein 1 (PD-1) inhibitor, was recently granted accelerated approval in advanced HCC. The CheckMate 040 trial (El-Khoueiry et al., 2017) looked at patients with HCC with or without HCV or HBV. Previous treatment with sorafenib was allowed, and patients did not need to have expression of programmed cell death-ligand 1. Results showed that in the 70% of patients previously treated with sorafenib, objective response was 16.2% in the dose-escalation cohort and 18.6% in the dose-expansion cohort (with complete responses achieved in each group). Very few patients were taken off the study because of toxicity. The safety profile was manageable and consistent across patient cohorts and was similar to what has been observed in other tumor types. Changes in endocrine and liver function were the most common adverse events. Prior to this study, sorafenib was the only treatment available for advanced-stage HCC. Currently, nivolumab is being compared to sorafenib as definitive treatment in patients with advanced HCC in the CheckMate 459 phase 3 study (NCCN, 2018).

Guidelines for Treatment

Cancer is the leading cause of death in women and men aged 60–79 years (NCCN, 2018). It is estimated that by 2030, approximately 70% of all cancers will be diagnosed in adults aged 65 years or older (Smith,

Smith, Hurria, Hortobagyi, & Buchholz, 2009). The increased longevity of the population means that a greater number of older adult patients with HCC are expected in the coming years (Nishikawa, Kimura, Kita, & Osaki, 2013). In the United States, HCC incidence peaks above the age of 70 years, and patients are most likely women and more likely to have HCV (Brunot, Le Sourd, Pracht, & Edeline, 2016; Nishikawa et al., 2013). As a result, HCC is a disease seen in older adults, with the small exception of those patients who may have genetic hemochromatosis. To date, results of most studies do not find any difference in terms of treatment outcomes between older adults and young patients, including studies comparing different treatments (Brunot et al., 2016).

Consequently, this population is at risk for being either undertreated, meaning the nondelivery of standard treatment due only to patients' age regardless of whether they are fit to receive it, or overtreated, meaning the administration of standard treatment despite the frailty of patients, which could cause severe toxicities or geriatric failure (Brunot et al., 2016). NCCN (2018) guidelines for older adult patients with cancer address specific issues related to the management of cancer in older adults, including performing screening and comprehensive geriatric assessment, assessing the risks and benefits of treatment, preventing and decreasing complications from therapy, and managing patients deemed to be at high risk for toxicity from standard treatment. Oncology nurses and providers should leverage these tools to be able to provide safe, quality care to older adults.

Clinical Trials Influencing Current Treatment

Many clinical trials are being conducted with patients with HCC. A clinical trial is also a good alternative to treatment because approved treatment options are limited in this population. New treatments may take longer to develop in this patient population because of the relatively few high-quality randomized clinical trials with hepatobiliary cancers. Patient participation in prospective clinical trials is the preferred option for the treatment of patients with all stages of this disease (NCCN, 2018). The areas being concentrated in clinical trials in patients with HCC include the adjuvant setting after resection and liver transplantation, combination treatments with sorafenib and immunotherapy in the advanced setting, and treatment after arterial therapy and radiation therapy. For a thorough list of current trials, healthcare providers and patients can refer to https://clinicaltrials.gov.

Nursing Care

Patients diagnosed with HCC have limited options and rely on information from many avenues to make treatment decisions. Oncology nurses are advocates for patients and can offer clinical trial information, provide supportive care, and be a liaison to providers to maximize patient outcomes.

Prognosis

The prognosis for HCC is variable and dependent on response and stage of disease (anatomic extension of the tumor) at presentation, performance status, and underlying liver function calculated using the Child-Pugh scoring system (described in the Treatment section). In general, the five-year survival rate for patients with liver cancer is 18% (ACS, 2018a). Forty-three percent of patients are diagnosed with localized disease, for which five-year survival is 31% (ACS, 2018a). Patients with advanced disease usually survive less than six months (NCI, 2018a).

Patients with early-stage disease are considered for curative treatment, which includes surgical resection, and have a five-year survival rate of 50%–75% (Ayuso et al., 2018). Patients with intermediate disease still have preserved liver function and HCC without vascular invasion or extrahepatic disease. Transarterial chemotherapy may lead to a four-year OS (Ayuso et al., 2018). Patients with a poor prognosis have the worst outcomes and usually die from liver failure.

In reference to treatment-related prognosis, the five-year OS rate for patients with early-stage HCC who are undergoing liver transplantation is 44%–78%; for those undergoing liver resection, the OS rate is 27%–70% (NCI, 2018a). At present, only 10%–23% of patients with HCC may be surgical candidates for curative-intent treatment (NCI, 2018a).

Prevention

Preventing sexually transmitted infections, such as hepatitis-related infections; avoiding excessive alcohol intake; and receiving vaccinations can assist in lowering a patient's risk of HCC. It is especially important to educate the adolescent population on these early primary preventive strategies. The high-risk population for contracting HBV are people receiving frequent blood transfusions, people receiving dialysis, solid organ transplant recipients, incarcerated individuals, illicit drug users, people with multiple sexual partners, healthcare workers, homosexual men, travelers to endemic areas, long-term facility residents, and patients with chronic liver disease, kidney disease, HIV, or diabetes. A vaccine that protects against HBV infection has been available since 1982. It is 95% effective in preventing infection and the development of chronic disease and liver cancer related to hepatitis B (Erb, 2018). However, no vaccine exists for HCV. If a patient already has hepatitis C, receiving early treatment with approved antivirals can lower a patient's chances of cirrhosis and thus lessen the chance of associated neoplasms.

Because of its link to obesity, nonalcoholic fatty liver disease is becoming an increasingly important risk factor for HCC. Maintaining a healthy weight, eating a balanced diet, and performing moderate physical activity at an early age can decrease risk and prevent disease. Taken all together, raising awareness for healthy food consumption, regulating obesity and diabetes, and limiting alcohol intake are valid approaches for prevention of HCC (Ozen & Dayanc, 2016).

High-Risk Assessment: Screening and Genetic Testing

The two hereditary genetic disorders associated with increased risk of HCC are genetic hemochromatosis and alpha-1 antitrypsin deficiency. Genetic hemochromatosis is a condition characterized by excess iron absorption due to the presence of mutations in the *HFE* gene. It is also a risk factor for HCC. A National Center for Health Statistics study found that patients with a known hemochromatosis diagnosis at death were 23 times more likely to have liver cancer than those without genetic hemochromatosis (NCCN, 2018). Genetic testing via cheek swab using whole blood can help diagnose genetic hemochromatosis. In contrast, alpha-1 antitrypsin deficiency is a hereditary genetic disorder that can lead to development of lung or liver disease. It is diagnosed by peripheral blood and results in low levels of alpha-1 antitrypsin in combination with abnormal liver function. Typically, patients with HCC are seen already with these diagnoses. Genetic testing is useful for patients wanting to have children so that they can be advised of the potential risks.

Surveillance

Surveillance recommendations for patients with HCC vary depending on the type of treatment received. For patients who are potentially surgically resectable or transplant eligible, or who have received a locoregional therapy, NCCN (2018) guidelines recommend imaging studies and AFP (if elevated) every 3–6 months for 2 years, then every 6–12 months thereafter. Hepatology should be included for antiviral therapy for carriers of hepatitis.

Survivorship

Although survivorship programs have been around for many years, it recently has been a rising topic in the forefront of post-treatment care, with many institutions having to meet accreditation requirements that ensure this care is available. However, these survivorship programs are limited to patients with stage I, II, and III disease. Because different staging systems can be used to stage HCC, it is difficult to categorize patients. However, NCI states that an individual is a cancer survivor from the time of diagnosis until the end of life ("Survivor," n.d.). Family members, friends, and caregivers are also affected by the survivorship experience and therefore are included in this definition. The journey for a patient with HCC starts at diagnosis and may have many roads and avenues due to uncertainty of response and liver function. For example, if they are candidates for a liver transplant, they may fear they will not receive the transplant in time. As a result, it is important for these patients and their caregivers to receive the needed support and resources from diagnosis and through post-treatment.

Patients in post-treatment, especially for those who received a liver transplant, have many survivorship concerns. They encounter many social, financial, and economic problems during this time. Additionally, secondary cancers are a risk. Risk of recurrence is also a very fearful topic for many patients. The recurrence rate after resection is approximately 50% in two years and 75% in five years (Sun et al., 2016). As a result, advanced practice providers should be cautious about when and how they present a survivorship program to patients with HCC. Patients should be educated on the purpose of survivorship care and prognosis, as this can cause heightened expectations regarding survival, depending on where patients are in their treatment. Survivorship care should be tailored to individuals' current and future needs. Despite the high recurrence rates, patients should be informed about the potential late effects of treatment (particularly cardiotoxicity effects) and also about surveillance. Referrals to the appropriate providers, especially allied healthcare providers, are important to keep in mind so that patients feel supported and engaged during the survivorship period.

Health education regarding preventive strategies, such as increasing physical activity, decreasing alcohol intake, eating a healthy diet, practicing safe sexual habits, adhering to medication instructions, and maintaining a healthy weight, is vital to improve overall health outcomes. Additionally, having a primary care physician available to care for the routine medical problems that may arise following treatment is critical to the continued care of cancer survivors. Primary care physicians should have a copy of the survivorship care plan so that they are aware of the late effects of treatments and long-term health risks associated with the previous cancer treatment. As nurses and providers, maintaining communication with the entire care team surrounding post-treatment care will assist in having good communication pathways that will benefit patients' survival outcomes and quality of life. Although some topics may entail areas that a nurse may not have knowledge of, it is important to provide the necessary resources so that patients can receive answers to difficult questions (Greenlee et al., 2016).

Biliary Tract Cancers: Cholangiocarcinoma and Gallbladder Cancer

Incidence and Epidemiology

The gallbladder is a small organ under the liver that concentrates and stores bile to aid in digestion. Gallbladder cancer is considered a rare cancer; 12,190 new diagnoses and 3,790 deaths were estimated for 2018 in the United States (ACS, 2018a). Gallbladder cancer is the fifth most common cancer involving the gastrointestinal tract (Rakić et al., 2014). Incidence rates are about 66% higher in women than in men (ACS, 2017). As mentioned, gallbladder cancer is considered a rare cancer of the digestive tract. A consortium from the European Union, the Surveillance of Rare Cancers in Europe (known as RARECARE), defined rare cancers as those with fewer than 6 cases per 100,000 people per year (ACS, 2017). On the other hand, gallbladder cancer is the most common malignancy of the biliary tract, representing 80%–95% of biliary tract cancers worldwide (Rakić et al., 2014). Outside of the United States (e.g., South America, India, Pakistan, Japan, Korea), the incidence of gallbladder cancer is higher because of the high prevalence of gallstones and chronic gallbladder infections (Recio-Boiles & Babiker, 2017).

Because of the rarity of these cancers, the statistics for cholangiocarcinoma also include gallbladder cancers, making it difficult to accurately estimate the number of cholangiocarcinoma cases. For 2018 in the United States, 54,410 new cases and 33,990 deaths were estimated by grouping liver, intrahepatic bile duct, gallbladder, and other biliary tract cancers (ACS, 2018a). These cancers can also be termed *hepatobiliary cancers*. As mentioned earlier, cholangiocarcinoma can be classified in subtypes: intrahepatic (perihilar) and extrahepatic. Extrahepatic cholangiocarcinomas occur more frequently than intrahepatic cholangiocarcinomas (NCCN, 2018).

Etiology and Risk Factors

The current hypothesis is that chronic inflammation of the bile duct tissues accumulates successive genomic mutations that lead to malignant transformation. The most common mutations described are the oncogenes *KRAS* and tumor suppression catenin beta 1 (*CTNNB1*) (Recio-Boiles & Babiker, 2017).

Chronic inflammation and bile stasis in the biliary tract are thought to be major risk factors underlying the pathogenesis of these cancers (Zhao & Lim, 2017). Gallstones are the highest risk factor, being present in most (85%) patients with gallbladder cancer, with larger stones causing more chronic inflammation and greater risk (Rakić et al., 2014).

Gallbladder cancer is often diagnosed at an advanced age, with 65% of patients older than 65 years (Goral, 2017). Because of its aggressive nature, the tumor can spread rapidly (NCCN, 2018). The risk is higher in women, people of Asian ethnicity, patients with a porcelain gallbladder (calcification of the gallbladder), and patients with chronic bacterial cholangitis (Rakić et al., 2014). Excess body weight has also been associated with gallbladder cancer. A recent study found that a 5 kg/m² increase in body mass index was associated with a 31% higher risk of gallbladder cancer (Bhaskaran et al., 2014). Other risk factors include anomalous pancreaticobiliary duct junctions, gallbladder polyps (solitary and symptomatic polyps larger than 1 cm), chronic typhoid infection, primary sclerosing cholangitis (PSC), and inflammatory bowel disease (Recio-Boiles & Babiker, 2017).

Cholangiocarcinoma generally occurs after the fourth decade of life. Aging is a risk factor, as is being of the male sex. Patients with PSC, which manifests in younger patients, is a risk factor. Other risk factors for cholangiocarcinoma are HCV infection, HBV infection, hepatolithiasis, abnormal pancreaticobiliary junction, choledochal cysts, nonalcoholic fatty liver disease, liver flukes, and tobacco use (Ebata et al., 2017).

Signs and Symptoms

Gallbladder cancers usually do not cause symptoms until the disease is in an advanced stage. Symptoms tend to be vague. Most patients are diagnosed after an elective cholecystectomy with confirmed pathology of malignancy. As a result, most patients present with symptoms typical to cholecystitis. The most common symptoms are persistent right upper quadrant pain, jaundice, nausea, and weight loss (Rakić et al., 2014). Other symptoms may include indigestion, weakness, general malaise, anorexia, and loss of appetite. This is also the case for patients with cholangiocarcinoma. Early-stage cholangiocarcinomas may manifest as only mild changes in serum liver function tests (NCCN, 2018).

Patients with PSC are at risk for cholangiocarcinoma and may not be diagnosed until late in the disease because of the overlapping disease of PSC that can make diagnosing cholangiocarcinoma more difficult. These patients often have frequent recurrent episodes of biliary obstruction and difficulties relieving obstructive jaundice. Biliary obstruction leads to clay-colored stools, amber-colored urine, and intense pruritus due to a lack of bile. More often than not, these patients have recurrent fevers related to the obstructive cholangitis. The presence of jaundice in patients with gallbladder cancer is usually associated with a poor prognosis. Patients with jaundice are more likely to have advanced disease (96% vs. 60%) and significantly lower disease-specific survival (6 months vs. 16 months) than patients without jaundice (Brandi, Venturi, Pantaleo, & Ercolani, 2016). Signs on physical examination at an advanced stage are abdominal pain, malaise, night sweats, and cachexia (Blechacz, 2017).

Diagnostic Evaluation

Diagnosis of biliary tract cancers can be challenging because of their anatomic location and late presentation. If obstructive jaundice is present, this can also contribute to the difficulty in obtaining a diagnosis. For initial workup, a complete abdominal ultrasound or CT scan usually is performed. These examinations typically are done to show the extent of biliary obstruction and to evaluate for conditions such as gallstones. Specifically, for gallbladder cancer, if gallstones are present combined with signs consistent for acute cholecystitis, then the patient may be referred for surgery without further workup. However, with a suspicion of a biliary or gallbladder cancer, consideration should be made to complete the staging examinations during the initial workup. High-quality, contrast-enhanced cross-sectional imaging (CT or MRI) of the chest, abdomen, and pelvis with IV contrast is recommended by NCCN (2018). This is to evaluate for tumor penetration through the wall of the gallbladder, the presence of nodal and distant metastases, and the extent of direct tumor invasion of other organs or major vascular invasion (NCCN, 2018). The same examinations are recommended for cholangiocarcinomas per NCCN. Additionally, for cholangiocarcinomas, imaging examinations are also important to assess the aforementioned and to determine the extent of liver involvement.

For patients presenting with jaundice, additional workup should include cholangiography to evaluate for hepatic and biliary invasion of tumor (NCCN, 2018). Magnetic resonance cholangiography and magnetic resonance angiography quite accurately detect bile duct or vascular invasion, with sensitivity and specificity approaching 100% (Rakić et al., 2014). Ideally, a magnetic resonance cholangiopancreatography should be performed before biliary drainage to avoid collapse of the biliary tree (Squadroni et al., 2017).

The role of PET-CT is still controversial, and it should be performed in specialized centers where small tumors can be detected (Squadroni et al., 2017). Of note, many false-positive PET scans can be seen when patients have obstructive jaundice, infection, or other sources of inflammation. As a result, PET is reserved for specific cases that are deemed appropriate by an interprofessional team.

Additionally, a complete blood count, complete metabolic panel including liver profile, and coagulation studies can be ordered. If bilirubin is elevated, coagulation may be affected, and attention should be given to these laboratory results because invasive procedures may be recommended.

Other tests to consider include tumor markers. The tumor marker related to biliary tract cancer is CA 19-9. Unfortunately, some patients do not express an elevated CA 19-9 biomarker. This is due to patients having negative undetectable Lewis antigen. As a result, it should not be relied on to diagnose a biliary tract cancer. CA 19-9 is also expressed in other malignancies and benign medical conditions. CA 19-9 has a sensitivity of 89% and a specificity of 86% even though levels may be affected by bile duct obstruction and acute cholangitis (Squadroni et al., 2017).

In practice, CA 19-9 levels should be assessed once patients have resolved the biliary obstruction. The biomarker carcinoembryonic antigen (known as CEA) can also be tested if CA 19-9 levels are undetectable, although it has a low predictive value (Squadroni et al., 2017). However, the biomarker CA 19-9 is useful in showing treatment response prior to restaging, in surveillance, and may assist in deciding on treatment changes if an unexpected rise is seen. Differentiating between intrahepatic cholangiocarcinoma and HCC can be difficult. AFP testing should be considered, especially if the patient has chronic liver disease. A number of mixed HCC/intrahepatic cholangiocarcinomas may also present with an elevated AFP (NCCN, 2018).

Obtaining the diagnosis of gallbladder cancer or a biliary duct cancer can be difficult. An endoscopic ultrasound is considered more accurate than ultrasound (76%) and is useful in the differential diagnosis to correctly detect histologic neoplasia (97%) (Recio-Boiles & Babiker, 2017). Other ways to obtain the diagnosis can be via bile cytology by fine needle aspiration with ultrasound or CT, brush cytology via endoscopic retrograde cholangiography, endoscopic ultrasound, transpapillary biopsy, or during a percutaneous transhepatic cholangiography. Patients during this time may exhibit feelings of anxiety and frustration due to the inability to obtain a tissue diagnosis and repeated procedures in attempts to obtain a diagnosis prior to undergoing chemotherapy or chemoradiation. For example, brush cytology in endoscopic retrograde cholangiography fails to demonstrate the disease in 50% of cases (Goral, 2017).

Histology

Gallbladder cancer histologic classifications include the following (NCI, 2018):
- Adenocarcinoma, not otherwise specified
- Adenocarcinoma, intestinal type
- Adenosquamous carcinoma
- Carcinoma in situ
- Clear cell adenocarcinoma
- Mucinous adenocarcinoma
- Other (specify)

- Papillary carcinoma
- Signet ring cell carcinoma
- Small cell carcinoma (oat cell)
- Spindle cell and giant cell types
- Undifferentiated carcinoma

For biliary tract cancers, intrahepatic cholangiocarcinoma includes the following histologic classifications:
- Mass-forming tumor growth pattern
- Periductal tumor growth pattern
- Mass-forming and periductal infiltrating growth pattern

For mixed hepatocellular cholangiocarcinoma, perihilar bile duct cancer and distal bile duct cancers include the following:
- Adenocarcinoma, not otherwise specified
- Adenocarcinoma, intestinal type
- Carcinoma in situ
- Carcinoma, not otherwise specified
- Clear cell adenocarcinoma
- Mucinous adenocarcinoma
- Papillary carcinoma, invasive
- Papillary carcinoma, noninvasive
- Papillomatosis
- Signet ring cell carcinoma
- Small cell carcinoma (oat cell)
- Small cell types
- Spindle cell and giant cell types
- Squamous cell carcinoma
- Undifferentiated carcinoma

Clinical Staging

An AJCC and Union for International Cancer Control 2017 group separated the staging systems of cholangiocarcinoma depending on the location of the bile duct cancer (i.e., perihilar, distal, and intrahepatic) (Recio-Boiles & Babiker, 2017). Gallbladder cancer also has a separate staging system per AJCC. Prognostic stage groups according to the AJCC TNM staging system are as follows:
- Gallbladder cancer (Zhu, Pawlik, Kooby, Schefter, & Vauthey, 2017)
  - Stage 0: Tis N0 M0
  - Stage I: T1 N0 M0
  - Stage IIA: T2a N0 M0
  - Stage IIB: T2b N0 M0
  - Stage IIIA: T3 N0 M0
  - Stage IIIB: T1–T3 N1 M0
  - Stage IVA: T4 N0–1 M0
  - Stage IVB: Any T, N2 M0 or Any T, Any N, M1

- Intrahepatic cholangiocarcinoma (Aloia, Pawlik, Taouli, Rubbia-Brandt, & Vauthey, 2017)
  - Stage 0: Tis N0 M0
  - Stage IA: T1a N0 M0
  - Stage IB: T1b N0 M0
  - Stage II: T2 N0 M0
  - Stage IIIA: T3 N0 M0
  - Stage IIIB: T4 N0 M0 or Any T, N1 M0
  - Stage IV: Any T, Any N, M1
- Distal extrahepatic cholangiocarcinoma (Krasinskas, Pawlik, Mino-Kenudson, & Vauthey, 2017)
  - Stage 0: Tis N0 M0
  - Stage I: T1 N0 M0
  - Stage IIA: T1 N1 M0 or T2 N0 M0
  - Stage IIB: T2 N1 M0, T3 N0 M0, or T3 N1 M0
  - Stage IIIA: T1 N2 M0, T2 N2 M0, or T3 N2 M0
  - Stage IIIB: T4 N0 M0, T4 N1 M0, or T4 N2 M0
  - Stage IV: Any T, Any N, M1
- Perihilar cholangiocarcinoma (Nagorney, Pawlik, Chun, Ebata, & Vauthey, 2017)
  - Stage 0: Tis N0 M0
  - Stage I: T1 N0 M0
  - Stage II: T2a–b N0 M0
  - Stage IIIA: T3 N0 M0
  - Stage IIIB: T4 N0 M0
  - Stage IIIC: Any T, N1 M0
  - Stage IVA: Any T, N2 M0
  - Stage IVB: Any T, Any N, M1

Treatment

Surgery

Surgery is the only potentially curative modality, but most patients are asymptomatic until late in the disease course and therefore present with locally advanced or metastatic disease (Zhao & Lim, 2017). Only 10%–15% of biliary tract cancers are amenable to surgery at initial presentation (Nathan et al., 2007). Patients with cholangiocarcinoma or gallbladder cancer should be offered surgical resection, which represents the only treatment associated with long-term survival and the possibility for cure. Achieving a tumor-free surgical margin, which forms one of the most robust prognostic indicators, is the primary goal of resection for these tumors (Ebata et al., 2017).

In reference to gallbladder cancer, resection may be needed if the initial surgery was only intended to remove the gallbladder for the diagnosis of cholecystitis. Surgery for gallbladder cancer consists of a cholecystectomy, en bloc liver resection, lymphadenectomy, and bile duct resection if necessary (Squadroni et al., 2017).

Depending on the anatomic location of the cholangiocarcinoma, several different types of surgical techniques can be performed. Distal lesions are treated with a pancreaticoduodenectomy (Whipple procedure), intrahepatic lesions will require a hepatectomy with lymphadenectomy, and techniques for hilar lesions will vary according to the Bismuth-Corlette anatomic classification (Recio-Boiles & Babiker, 2018).

Transplant surgery in the case of unresectable hilar cholangiocarcinoma is still investigational and performed only in experienced centers. However, available data exist that support liver transplantation in selected cases of hilar cholangiocarcinoma—such as those not suitable for liver resection for local extension, or cirrhosis, but without nodal or metastatic involvement (Squadroni et al., 2017). Findings regarding the role of liver transplantation in intrahepatic cholangiocarcinoma are still controversial because of small sample sizes and the heterogeneity of perioperative treatment (adjuvant, neoadjuvant) (Squadroni et al., 2017).

Preoperative management: During the preoperative period, patients may need to undergo additional workup. A diagnostic laparoscopy may be performed to ensure there is no evidence of metastatic disease prior to undergoing surgery. Additionally, laboratory work, anesthesia clearance (including cardiology and respiratory examinations), and evaluation of coagulation problems should be addressed. Preoperative biliary drainage and accurate clinical evaluation may be considered because extended surgical resection and lymphadenectomy have a high risk for perioperative morbidity (Squadroni et al., 2017). Additionally, a portal vein embolization may be recommended for patients with borderline liver function to achieve liver hypertrophy to the opposite side of the liver. An interventional radiologist typically performs this procedure at least four to six weeks prior to surgery to allow sufficient time for liver hypertrophy. Timing is critical when having multiple staged procedures. Therefore, all interprofessional team members must be aware of each time point so that the opportunity for resection is not lost.

Patients should receive education on the typical length of time of the procedure, length of hospital stay, and possible postoperative complications. It also is possible that the surgery will be aborted intraoperatively if the tumor is found to be unresectable. Ensuring awareness of this ahead of time will provide patients and their caregivers the understanding that surgery may not be definitive despite the staging workup.

Similar to patients undergoing resection for HCC, the preoperative time is marked by anxiety because of the waiting time between the first visit and the surgery. During this time, an interprofessional team will evaluate and revaluate the patient's case to determine timing of surgery. Reassuring patients and providing continuous communication that precautions are being taken to ultimately improve their safety and outcomes during surgery will offer some relief to patients and their caregivers.

Postoperative management: Postsurgical outcomes and postoperative management are similar to those of patients with HCC, as discussed previously. Patients also are at risk for bile leaks. This is a critical time with frequent monitoring of liver function tests, and unusual increases in values should be reported immediately. Other signs that should be noted in order to prevent worsening of postsurgical complications are painless jaundice, amber-colored urine, and clay-colored stools.

Additional laboratory values that are monitored include coagulation studies and pancreatic enzymes (amylase and lipase). Many patients may have a Jackson-Pratt drain. Pancreatic enzymes, specifically amylase, will be monitored from the drain and compared to the serum levels. A pancreatic leak is identified on postoperative day 3 if the drain amylase is three times the serum amylase. Depending on the results, drains may be removed or kept in place. Drains with a pancreatic leak will be kept in place on discharge and then removed in the outpatient setting. Educating patients on the care and maintenance of drainage systems will help providers to determine the timing of removal.

Intake and output will also need to be monitored by nurses and patients during the postoperative period to prevent electrolyte imbalances, nutritional complications, and dehydration. Some patients may require a nasogastric tube to allow for stomach decompression and may be supported with total parenteral nutrition including lipids during the initial days to weeks postoperatively.

Increasing physical activity will assist in the prevention of a thromboembolic event and hospital-acquired pneumonia. Monitoring for possible infections is critical to the patient's recovery. This is done by reporting fevers and elevated white blood cell counts.

Communication regarding postdischarge care is one of the most important and overlooked areas in the postoperative period. Depending on the intraoperative findings and preliminary pathology, coordination of postsurgical care at home will be critical for patients to be able to continue their recovery and to consider treatment with other modalities such as chemotherapy or chemoradiation in the adjuvant setting. Initiating adjuvant treatment after surgery has been found to be most effective four to eight weeks after surgery. It is essential to ensure that a postsurgical follow-up appointment and a medical oncology appointment have been secured prior to discharge to avoid delays in treatment (Kapritsou et al., 2014).

Chemotherapy

Advances in the treatment of biliary tract cancers have been rare. Unfortunately, most of the data come from phase 2 trials or extrapolation of data from studies of patients with advanced disease. Accrual for clinical trials in biliary tract cancers is difficult because of the low number of diagnosed patients and the rarity of these cancers.

Retrospective studies combining gallbladder cancer and cholangiocarcinoma have provided conflicting evidence on the role of adjuvant therapy (NCCN, 2018). Many oncology physicians believe that cholangiocarcinomas should be separated from gallbladder cancers because of the differences in their biology. Like pancreatic cancer, even with curative resection, the risk of recurrence remains high. No definitive standard has been established in the adjuvant treatment of biliary tract cancers. Treatment options include fluoropyrimidine chemoradiation followed by additional fluoropyrimidine-based or gemcitabine chemotherapy, or fluoropyrimidine-based or gemcitabine-based chemotherapy for patients with positive regional nodes (NCCN, 2018).

In the advanced or metastatic setting, the chemotherapy regimen approved with category 1 evidence per NCCN is gemcitabine and cisplatin (NCCN, 2018). A clinical trial should always be considered in this population because of the lack of approved regimens and small benefits seen in survival from the standard-of-care treatments. Based on experiences from phase 2 studies, as of 2017, the following gemcitabine-based and fluoropyrimidine-based combination chemotherapy regimens are included with NCCN category 2A recommendation for treatment of patients with advanced biliary tract cancer: gemcitabine with oxaliplatin or capecitabine; capecitabine with cisplatin or oxaliplatin; 5-fluorouracil with cisplatin or oxaliplatin; and single-agent 5-fluorouracil, capecitabine, and gemcitabine (NCCN, 2018).

The nursing role comprises the early assessment of side effects, management of symptoms, and advocacy for palliative care when recommended. With the aforementioned regimens, side effects such as peripheral neuropathy, diarrhea, and myelosuppression occur most commonly. Some patients may not understand the rationale for holding treatment and may believe it will cause detriment to their response. A thorough discussion between the nurse and patient concerning this topic may ease the anxiety of missing a treatment. Patients may also present with portal hypertension, which can cause splenomegaly and, as a result, cause providers to hesitate in treating because of the threat of thrombocytopenia. These patients may require a splenic embolization to continue treatment. Additionally, educating patients on adherence to oral treatments will assist in optimizing their response to treatment and, hence, their quality of life. Supportive and palliative care measures should be considered to assist patients in continuing treatment.

Radiation Therapy

Data supporting particular chemoradiation and chemotherapy regimens for adjuvant treatment of resected biliary tract cancers are limited (NCCN, 2018). One phase 2 trial, SWOG S0809, shows promising results in the adjuvant setting, but phase 3 confirmation is still pending results. Results from the phase 2 trial showed two-year OS of 65% and median survival of 35 months (Ben-Josef et al., 2015). Of note, the trial enrolled patients with extrahepatic cholangiocarcinoma and gallbladder cancer (Ben-Josef et al., 2015). NCCN (2018) suggests using EBRT with three-dimensional conformal radiation and intensity-modulated radiation therapy as treatment options. Most of the collective experience of chemoradiation in biliary tract cancers involved concurrent chemoradiation with 5-fluorouracil as a sensitizing agent, as well as capecitabine (NCCN, 2018). Chemoradiation with gemcitabine is not recommended, because of limited experience and the toxicity associated with this treatment (NCCN, 2018). This same recommendation applies to the advanced setting. Chemoradiation in the setting of advanced biliary tract cancers can provide control of symptoms due to local tumor effects and may prolong OS (NCCN, 2018).

Nursing care of patients undergoing radiation includes education about the timing of radiation and the different phases of preparation (i.e., planning and simulation) prior to starting treatment, as the time leading up to treatment may be delayed. When adding chemotherapy to radiation, side effects such as diarrhea, mucositis, myelosuppression, and skin changes may arise. Providing detailed education on potential side effects and whom to contact will allow patients to feel supported through treatment, especially if the treatment is for curative intent.

Immunotherapy

Immunotherapy is making an impact in many cancers. Studies have indicated that mismatch repair–deficient (dMMR) tumors are sensitive to PD-1 blockade. Results were recently published from a study of patients with dMMR tumors of various sites. Among four patients with dMMR cholangiocarcinoma who received pembrolizumab, one patient had a complete response and the remaining had stable disease (Le et al., 2017). As a result, NCCN (2018) has included pembrolizumab as a treatment option for patients with unresectable or metastatic microsatellite instability–high/dMMR biliary tract tumors but cautions that data to support this recommendation are limited, particularly in the first-line setting. As of the time of this writing, ongoing clinical trials in this area are still being investigated, particularly in the phase 1 setting with single or double immunotherapy combinations.

Guidelines for Treatment

Biliary tract cancer is a disease of older adults, with the small exception of those patients who may have a familial history or a history of PSC. NCCN (2018) has developed guidelines on the care of older adult patients with cancer to ensure that a comprehensive geriatric assessment is performed in this population. Other assessments are also recommended, such as functional status, comorbidities, cognitive function, nutritional status, polypharmacy, medication review, psychological status, and social support. As a result, the focus is placed not on age but on clinical status, and all types of treatments for biliary tract cancer—surgery, chemotherapy, radiation therapy, and clinical trials—can be considered.

Clinical Trials Influencing Current Treatment

Clinical trials for patients with biliary tract cancer are uncommon because of the low number of patients diagnosed. As mentioned previously, gallbladder cancer and cholangiocarcinomas are grouped together in clinical trials. Limited trials occur in the adjuvant setting, but many ongoing trials in the advanced and metastatic setting are looking to either improve first-line treatment or obtain a second-line treatment that has better outcomes than the current NCCN category 2A treatment options. A clinical trial is also a good alternative because limited approved treatment options are available in this setting. However, significant statistical results will take time to become available because of the small number of patients diagnosed. For a thorough list of current trials, healthcare providers and patients can refer to https://clinicaltrials.gov.

The use of precision medicine in this arena has also become an avenue that providers can use to tailor treatments to biomarkers present in patients' individual cancer cells. Trastuzumab is a monoclonal antibody targeting HER2, and HER2 overexpression has been described in cholangiocarcinoma (Sorscher, 2014). However, only about 5% of biliary tract cancers overexpress HER2 (Sorscher, 2014). Phase 2 studies are ongoing at the time of this writing to investigate HER2-directed treatment options for solid tumors (NCCN, 2018).

Nursing Care

Patients diagnosed with biliary tract cancers have limited options, and patients rely on information from many avenues to make treatment decisions. Oncology nurses are advocates for patients and can offer information on clinical trials, provide supportive care, and be a liaison to providers to maximize patient outcomes.

Prognosis

The prognosis of gallbladder cancer is poor because of aggressive tumor biology, late presentation, complicated anatomic position, and advanced stage at diagnosis. Based on data from 10,000 patients diagnosed with gallbladder cancer from 1989 to 1996, the five-year survival rates started at 80% for stage 0, then progressively fell to 50% for stage I, 28% for stage II, 8% for stage IIIA, 7% for stage IIIB, 4% for stage IVA, and 2% for stage IVB (Edge et al., 2010).

Cholangiocarcinoma is rare and highly lethal because of the locally advanced unresectable stage at diagnosis (Recio-Boiles & Babiker, 2018). Prognosis is poor, with five-year survival rates of 20%–50% after resection and almost 0% in unresectable tumors. However, knowledge of tumor biology has increased and, combined with nonsurgical management, has resulted in improved outcomes. Aggressive surgical approaches have resulted in R0 resections, but recurrence rates are 49%–64% (Blechacz, 2017). Recurrences are intrahepatic and occur within two to three years (Blechacz, 2017). Five-year survival rates are 10% for stage 3 and 0% for stage 4 (Brandi et al., 2016). Death is often caused by biliary sepsis, cancer cachexia, malnutrition, and liver failure (National Institutes of Health Genetic and Rare Diseases Information Center, 2012).

Prevention

For patients with PSC, bile duct brush cytologic examination or biopsy may be used as surveillance for early detection of cellular atypia (Squadroni et al., 2017). Additionally, prevention of sexually transmitted infections, such as hepatitis-related infections; vaccinations; and avoidance of excessive alcohol intake can assist in lowering the risk of biliary tract cancers. For patients who already have hepatitis, early treatment can lower their chances of cirrhosis and hence lessen the chance of associated neoplasms.

High-Risk Assessment: Screening and Genetic Testing

Most bile duct cancers are not found in people with a family history of this disease. Inherited gene mutations are not thought to cause many bile duct cancers; therefore, it is rare to refer patients to genetic testing. Hereditary nonpolyposis colorectal cancer syndrome can increase the risk for a biliary or liver cancer. In general, these patients have an extensive family and personal history of cancer and are diagnosed at a younger age. Despite the greater than ninefold increased risk of bile duct cancer in patients with hereditary nonpolyposis colorectal cancer syndrome, routine screening for bile duct cancers has not been recommended, owing in large part to the difficulty in detecting these cancers and their rarity (Haddad, Kowdley, Pawlik, & Cunningham, 2011).

Surveillance

Surveillance of patients with cancer in this population is recommended after treatment has been completed (i.e., either after surgical resection with or without adjuvant therapy). NCCN (2018) guidelines recommend that follow-up of patients undergoing resection of cholangiocarcinoma and gallbladder cancer include consideration of imaging studies every six months for two years, then annually up to five years. Imaging examinations that can be considered during surveillance are a multiphasic abdominal/pelvic CT or MRI with IV contrast and a chest CT with or without contrast. Additionally, tumor marker testing can be performed with timing of imaging examinations for correlation of results.

Survivorship

Although survivorship programs have been around for many years, survivorship has become a rising topic in the forefront of post-treatment care. Many institutions have had to develop a survivorship program to meet accreditation requirements. The role of oncology nurses after completion of primary treatment is still emerging, as are models for delivering specific elements of long-term survivorship care in primary care and oncology settings (Klemp, Frazier, Glennon, Trunecek, & Irwin, 2011).

Survivorship issues for patients with biliary tract cancer are similar to those for patients with pancreatic cancer. Discussing survivorship with patients with biliary tract cancer, who have a very high risk of recurrence even after curative intent, is difficult. The recurrence rates remain as high as 50%–60% (Zhao & Lim, 2017). As a result, structured survivorship programs and knowledge on survivorship are lacking within this population. Physicians and advanced practice providers should be cautious when presenting a survivorship program to patients with biliary tract cancer. Patients should be educated on the purpose of survivorship care, as it can cause heightened expectations regarding survival. Despite the dismal prognosis and recurrence rates for this disease, patients should be educated after treatment on important survivorship issues, such as late effects of treatment (particularly peripheral neuropathy) and surveillance. Other areas that may need to be addressed include physical challenges, mental and emotional challenges, and financial and economic challenges. Referrals to the appropriate providers, especially allied healthcare providers, are important so that these patients feel supported and engaged during the survivorship period (Greenlee et al., 2016).

Health education regarding preventive strategies, such as increasing physical activity and maintaining a healthy weight, is important to decrease recurrence risk. Additionally, having a primary care physician available to care for the routine medical problems that may arise during the post-treatment period is critical to the continued care of cancer survivors. Primary care physicians should have a copy of the survivorship care plan so that they are aware of the late effects of treatments and long-term health risks associated with the previous cancer treatment. As nurses and providers, maintaining communication with the entire care team surrounding post-treatment care will assist in having good communication pathways that will benefit patients' survival outcomes and quality of life. Although some topics may entail areas that a nurse may not have knowledge of, it is important to provide the necessary resources so that patients can receive answers to difficult questions (Greenlee et al., 2016).

Summary

HCC incidence rates continue to increase, although mortality continues to decrease. Surgery is the only curative option but is no longer the first-line treatment of this cancer, as locoregional therapies are now included. New chemotherapy agents have been developed that have shown the ability to prevent disease progression. Disease control is the goal of HCC treatment. Surveillance is imperative to aggressively treat new recurrences. Survivorship programs can help patients cope with the side effects of treatment.

More than 65% of patients with cholangiocarcinoma have nonresectable disease at the time of diagnosis, resulting in a poor prognosis (Brandi et al., 2016). For unresectable intrahepatic cholangiocarcinoma, survival is three to six months (Brandi et al., 2016). Because cholangiocarcinoma is a rare cancer, referral to a cancer center is preferred because of the availability of an interprofessional team. Surgery is the only potential curative treatment.

References

Abou-Alfa, G.K., Pawlik, T.M., Shindoh, J., & Vauthey, J.-N. (2017). Liver. In M.B. Amin (Ed.), *AJCC cancer staging manual* (8th ed., pp. 287–293). Chicago, IL: Springer.

Ahn, D.H., & Bekaii-Saab, T. (2017). Biliary cancer: Intrahepatic cholangiocarcinoma vs. extrahepatic cholangiocarcinoma vs. gallbladder cancers: Classification and therapeutic implications. *Journal of Gastrointestinal Oncology, 8,* 293–301. https://doi.org/10.21037/jgo.2016.10.01

Aloia, T., Pawlik, T.M., Taouli, B., Rubbia-Brandt, L., & Vauthey, J.-N. (2017). Intrahepatic bile ducts. In M.B. Amin (Ed.), *AJCC cancer staging manual* (8th ed., pp. 295–302). Chicago, IL: Springer.

American Cancer Society. (n.d.). Bile duct cancer. Retrieved from https://www.cancer.org/cancer/bile-duct-cancer.html

American Cancer Society. (2016, April 28). Liver cancer risk factors. Retrieved from https://www.cancer.org/cancer/liver-cancer/causes-risks-prevention/risk-factors.html

American Cancer Society. (2017). Special section: Rare cancers in adults. Retrieved from https://www.cancer.org/content/dam/cancer-org/research/cancer-facts-and-statistics/annual-cancer-facts-and-figures/2017/cancer-facts-and-figures-2017-special-section-rare-cancers-in-adults.pdf

American Cancer Society. (2018a). *Cancer facts and figures 2018*. Retrieved from https://www.cancer.org/content/dam/cancer-org/research/cancer-facts-and-statistics/annual-cancer-facts-and-figures/2018/cancer-facts-and-figures-2018.pdf

American Cancer Society. (2018b, January 4). Key statistics about liver cancer. Retrieved from https://www.cancer.org/cancer/liver-cancer/about/what-is-key-statistics.html

Ayuso, C., Rimola, J., Vilana, R., Burrel, M., Darnell, A., García-Criado, A., ... Brú, C. (2018). Diagnosis and staging of hepatocellular carcinoma (HCC): Current guidelines. *European Journal of Radiology, 101,* 72–81. https://doi.org/10.1016/j.ejrad.2018.01.025

Ben-Josef, E., Guthrie, K.A., El-Khoueiry, A.B., Corless, C.L., Zalupski, M.M., Lowy, A.M., ... Blanke, C.D. (2015). SWOG S0809: A phase II intergroup trial of adjuvant capecitabine and gemcitabine followed by radiotherapy and concurrent capecitabine in extrahepatic and gallbladder carcinoma. *Journal of Clinical Oncology, 33,* 2617–2622. https://doi.org/10.1200/JCO.2014.60.2219

Benson, A.B., III, D'Angelica, M.I., Abbott, D.E., Abrams, T.A., Alberts, S.R., Anaya, D.A., ... Darlow, S. (2017). NCCN Guidelines Insights: Hepatobiliary cancers, version 1.2017. *Journal of the National Comprehensive Cancer Network, 15,* 563–573. https://doi.org/10.6004/jnccn.2017.0059

Bhaskaran, K., Douglas, I., Forbes, H., dos-Santos-Silva, I., Leon, D.A., & Smeeth, L. (2014). Body-mass index and risk of 22 specific cancers: A population-based cohort of 5.24 million UK adults. *Lancet, 384,* 755–765. https://doi.org/10.1016/S0140-6736(14)60892-8.

Blechacz, B. (2017). Cholangiocarcinoma: Current knowledge and new developments. *Gut and Liver, 11,* 13–26. https://doi.org/10.5009/gnl15568

Brandi, G., Venturi, M., Pantaleo, M.A., & Ercolani, G. (2016). Cholangiocarcinoma: Current opinion on clinical practice diagnostic and therapeutic algorithms. A review of the literature and a long-standing experience of a referral center. *Digestive and Liver Disease, 48,* 231–241. https://doi.org/10.1016/j.dld.2015.11.017

Bruix, J., Qin, S., Merle, P., Granito, A., Huang, Y.-H., Bodoky, G., ... Han, G. (2017). Regorafenib for patients with hepatocellular carcinoma who progressed on sorafenib treatment (RESORCE): A randomised, double-blind, placebo-controlled, phase 3 trial. *Lancet, 389,* 56–66. https://doi.org/10.1016/S0140-6736(16)32453-9

Bruix, J., Reig, M., & Sherman, M. (2016). Evidence-based diagnosis, staging, and treatment of patients with hepatocellular carcinoma. *Gastroenterology, 150,* 835–853. https://doi.org/10.1053/j.gastro.2015.12.041

Brunot, A., Le Sourd, S., Pracht, M., & Edeline, J. (2016). Hepatocellular carcinoma in elderly patients: Challenges and solutions. *Journal of Hepatocellular Carcinoma, 3,* 9–18. https://doi.org/10.2147/JHC.S101448

Cancer.Net. (2017, May). Liver cancer: Diagnosis. Retrieved from https://www.cancer.net/cancer-types/liver-cancer/diagnosis

Dutta, R., & Mahato, R.I. (2017). Recent advances in hepatocellular carcinoma therapy. *Pharmacology and Therapeutics, 173,* 106–117. https://doi.org/10.1016/j.pharmthera.2017.02.010

Ebata, T., Ercolani, G., Alvaro, D., Ribero, D., Di Tommaso, L., & Valle, J.W. (2017). Current status on cholangiocarcinoma and gallbladder cancer. *Liver Cancer, 6,* 59–65. https://doi.org/10.1159/000449493

Edge, S.B., Byrd, D.R., Compton, C.C., Fritz, A.G., Greene, F.L., & Trotti, A., III. (Eds.). (2010). *AJCC cancer staging manual* (7th ed.). Chicago, IL: Springer.

El-Khoueiry, A.B., Sangro, B., Yau, T., Crocenzi, T.S., Kudo, M., Hsu, C., ... Melero, I. (2017). Nivolumab in patients with advanced hepatocellular carcinoma (CheckMate

040): An open-label, non-comparative, phase 1/2 dose escalation and expansion trial. *Lancet, 389,* 2492–2502. https://doi.org/10.1016/S0140-6736(17)31046-2

Erb, C.H. (2018). Viruses and vaccines. In J.L. Watson (Ed.), *Your guide to cancer prevention* (pp. 93–106). Pittsburgh, PA: Oncology Nursing Society.

Goral, V. (2017). Cholangiocarcinoma: New insights. *Asian Pacific Journal of Cancer Prevention, 18,* 1469–1473. https://doi.org/10.22034/APJCP.2017.18.6.1469

Greenlee, H., Molmenti, C.L.S., Crew, K.D., Awad, D., Kalinsky, K., Brafmen, L., ... Hershman, D.L. (2016). Survivorship care plans and adherence to lifestyle recommendations among breast cancer survivors. *Journal of Cancer Survivorship, 10,* 956–963. https://doi.org/10.1007/s11764-016-0541-8

Haddad, A., Kowdley, G.C., Pawlik, T.M., & Cunningham, S.C. (2011). Hereditary pancreatic and hepatobiliary cancers. *International Journal of Surgical Oncology, 2011,* 1–10. https://doi.org/10.1155/2011/154673

Holzwanger, D.J., & Madoff, D.C. (2018). Role of interventional radiology in the management of hepatocellular carcinoma: Current status. *Chinese Clinical Oncology.* Advance online publication. https://doi.org/10.21037/cco.2018.07.04

Kapritsou, M., Korkolis, D.P., Giannakopoulou, M., Kaklamanos, I., Elefsiniotis, I.S., Mariolis-Sapsakos, T., ... Konstantinou, E.A. (2014). Fast-track recovery after major liver and pancreatic resection from the nursing point of view. *Gastroenterology Nursing, 37,* 228–233. https://doi.org/10.1097/SGA.0000000000000049

Klemp, J.R., Frazier, L.M., Glennon, C., Trunecek, J., & Irwin, M. (2011). Improving cancer survivorship care: Oncology nurses' educational needs and preferred methods of learning. *Journal of Cancer Education, 26,* 234–242. https://doi.org/10.1007/s13187-011-0193-3

Krasinskas, A., Pawlik, T.M., Mino-Kenudson, M., & Vauthey, J.-N. (2017). Distal bile duct. In M.B. Amin (Ed.), *AJCC cancer staging manual* (8th ed., pp. 317–325). Chicago, IL: Springer.

Le, D.T., Durham, J.N., Smith, K.N., Wang, H., Bartlett, B.R., Aulakh, L.K., ... Diaz, L.A., Jr. (2017). Mismatch repair deficiency predicts response of solid tumors to PD-1 blockade. *Science, 357,* 409–413. https://doi.org/10.1126/science.aan6733

Llovet, J.M., Ricci, S., Mazzaferro, V., Hilgard, P., Gane, E., Blanc, J.-F., ... Bruix, J. (2008). Sorafenib in advanced hepatocellular carcinoma. *New England Journal of Medicine, 359,* 378–390. https://doi.org/10.1056/NEJMoa0708857

Marrero, J.A., Kulik, L.M., Sirlin, C.B., Zhu, A.X., Finn, R.S., Abecassis, M.M., ... Heimbach, J.K. (2018). Diagnosis, staging, and management of hepatocellular carcinoma: 2018 practice guidance by the American Association for the Study of Liver Diseases. *Hepatology, 68,* 723–750. https://doi.org/10.1002/hep.29913

Nagorney, D.M., Pawlik, T.M., Chun, Y.S., Ebata, T., & Vauthey, J.-N. (2017). Perihilar bile ducts. In M.B. Amin (Ed.), *AJCC cancer staging manual* (8th ed., pp. 311–316). Chicago, IL: Springer.

Nathan, H., Pawlik, T.M., Wolfgang, C.L., Choti, M.A., Cameron, J.L., & Schulik, R.D. (2007). Trends in survival after surgery for cholangiocarcinoma: A 30-year population-based SEER database analysis. *Journal of Gastrointestinal Surgery, 11,* 1488–1497.

National Cancer Institute. (2018a, February 6). Adult primary liver cancer treatment (PDQ®) [Health professional version]. Retrieved from https://www.cancer.gov/types/liver/hp/adult-liver-treatment-pdq

National Cancer Institute. (2018b, July 5). Bile duct cancer (cholangiocarcinoma) treatment (PDQ®) [Patient version]. Retrieved from https://www.cancer.gov/types/liver/patient/bile-duct-treatment-pdq

National Cancer Institute. (2018c, March 22). Gallbladder cancer treatment (PDQ®) [Patient version]. Retrieved from https://www.cancer.gov/types/gallbladder/patient/gallbladder-treatment-pdq

National Comprehensive Cancer Network. (2018). *NCCN Clinical Practice Guidelines in Oncology (NCCN Guidelines®): Hepatobiliary cancers* [v.4.2018]. Retrieved from https://www.nccn.org/professionals/physician_gls/pdf/hepatobiliary.pdf

National Institutes of Health Genetic and Rare Diseases Information Center. (2012, September). Bile duct cancer. Retrieved from https://rarediseases.info.nih.gov/diseases/9304/index

Nishikawa, H., Kimura, T., Kita, R., & Osaki, Y. (2013). Treatment for hepatocellular carcinoma in elderly patients: A literature review. *Journal of Cancer, 4,* 635–643. https://doi.org/10.7150/jca.7279

Ozen, C., & Dayanc, B.E. (2016). Current prevention approaches for hepatocellular carcinoma. *Journal of Cancer Prevention and Current Research, 4*(1), 1–3. https://doi.org/10.15406/jcpcr.2016.04.00103

Qin, S., Bai, Y., Lim, H.Y., Thongprasert, S., Chao, Y., Fan, J., ... Sun, Y. (2013). Randomized, multicenter, open-label study of oxaliplatin plus fluorouracil/leucovorin versus doxorubicin as palliative chemotherapy in patients with advanced hepatocellular carcinoma from Asia. *Journal of Clinical Oncology, 31,* 3501–3508. https://doi.org/10.1200/JCO.2012.44.5643

Rakić, M., Patrlj, L., Kopljar, M., Kliček, R., Kolovrat, M., Loncar, B., & Busic, Z. (2014). Gallbladder cancer. *Hepatobiliary Surgery and Nutrition, 3,* 221–226. https://doi.org/10.3978/j.issn.2304-3881.2014.09.03

Recio-Boiles, A., & Babiker, H.M. (2017, October 6). Cancer, gallbladder. Retrieved from https://www.ncbi.nlm.nih.gov/books/NBK442002

Recio-Boiles, A., & Babiker, H.M. (2018, September 17). Cancer, hepatobiliary tract. Retrieved from https://www.ncbi.nlm.nih.gov/books/NBK441830

Ryerson, A.B., Eheman, C.R., Altekruse, S.F., Ward, J.W., Jemal, A., Sherman, R.L., ... Kohler, B.A. (2016). Annual report to the nation on the status of cancer, 1975–2012, featuring the increasing incidence of liver cancer. *Cancer, 122,* 1312–1337. https://doi.org/10.1002/cncr.29936

Sadati, L., Pazouki, A., Mehdizadeh, A., Shoar, S., Tamannaie, Z., & Chaichian, S. (2013). Effect of preoperative nursing visit on preoperative anxiety and postoperative complications in candidates for laparoscopic cholecystectomy: A randomized clinical trial. *Scandinavian Journal of Caring Sciences, 27,* 994–998. https://doi.org/10.1111/scs.12022

Sanyal, A.J., Yoon, S.K., & Lencioni, R. (2010). The etiology of hepatocellular carcinoma and consequences for treatment. *Oncologist, 15*(Suppl. 4), 14–22. https://doi.org/10.1634/theoncologist.2010-S4-14

Sapisochin, G., & Bruix, J. (2017). Liver transplantation for hepatocellular carcinoma: Outcomes and novel surgical approaches. *Nature Reviews Gastroenterology and Hepatology, 14,* 203–217. https://doi.org/10.1038/nrgastro.2016.193

Smith, B.D., Smith, G.L., Hurria, A., Hortobagyi, G.N., & Buchholz, T.A. (2009). Future of cancer incidence in the United States: Burdens upon an aging, changing nation. *Journal of Clinical Oncology, 27,* 2758–2765. https://doi.org/10.1200/JCO.2008.20.8983

Sorscher, S. (2014). Marked radiographic response of a HER-2-overexpressing biliary cancer to trastuzumab. *Cancer Management and Research, 2014*(6), 1–3. https://doi.org/10.2147/CMAR.S55091

Squadroni, M., Tondulli, L., Gatta, G., Mosconi, S., Beretta, G., & Labianca, R. (2017). Cholangiocarcinoma. *Critical Reviews in Oncology/Hematology, 116,* 11–31. https://doi.org/10.1016/j.critrevonc.2016.11.012

Subramaniam, S., Kelley, R.K., & Venook, A.P. (2013). A review of hepatocellular carcinoma (HCC) staging systems. *Chinese Clinical Oncology, 2*(4), 33. https://doi.org/10.3978/j.issn.2304-3865.2013.07.05

Sun, D.-W., An, L., Wei, F., Mu, L., Shi, X.-J., Wang, C.-L., ... Lv, G.-Y. (2016). Prognostic significance of parameters from pretreatment ^{18}F-FDG PET in hepatocellular carcinoma: A meta-analysis. *Abdominal Radiology, 41,* 33–41. https://doi.org/10.1007/s00261-015-0603-9

Sur, B.W., & Sharma, A. (2018). Transarterial chemoembolization for hepatocellular carcinoma. *Journal of Radiology Nursing, 37,* 107–111. https://doi.org/10.1016/j.jradnu.2017.12.004

Survivor. (n.d.). In *NCI dictionary of cancer terms.* Retrieved from https://www.cancer.gov/publications/dictionaries/cancer-terms/def/survivor

Wang, C.-H., Wey, K.-C., Mo, L.-R., Chang, K.-K., Lin, R.-C., & Kuo, J.-J. (2015). Current trends and recent advances in diagnosis, therapy, and prevention of hepatocellular carcinoma. *Asian Pacific Journal of Cancer Prevention, 16,* 3595–3604. https://doi.org/10.7314/APJCP.2015.16.9.3595

Zhao, D.Y., & Lim, K.-H. (2017). Current biologics for treatment of biliary tract cancers. *Journal of Gastrointestinal Oncology, 8,* 430–440. https://doi.org/10.21037/jgo.2017.05.04

Zhu, A.X., Pawlik, T.M., Kooby, D.A., Schefter, T.E., & Vauthey, J.-N. (2017). Gallbladder. In M.B. Amin (Ed.), *AJCC cancer staging manual* (8th ed., pp. 303–309). Chicago, IL: Springer.

CHAPTER 7

Small Bowel Cancer

*Jessica MacIntyre, ARNP, NP-C, AOCNP®, and
Amber Thomassen, MA, MSN, APRN-BC, AOCNP®*

Introduction

According to the American Cancer Society (ACS, 2018d), small bowel cancers are made up of cells that grow out of control in this portion of the gastrointestinal (GI) tract. The small intestine is responsible for continued food breakdown and absorption of most of the nutrients. The small intestine has three sections (see Figure 7-1). The first is the shortest and is known as the duodenum. It is where the contents of the stomach are emptied. The second and third sections are the jejunum and ileum, which absorb nutrients from digested food into the bloodstream (ACS, 2018d). Tumors that arise in the small intestine can be benign or malignant (Mayer, 2017).

Incidence and Epidemiology

In the United States, 10,470 new cases of small bowel cancer and 1,450 deaths were estimated for 2018 (Siegel, Miller, & Jemal, 2018). Although the small bowel comprises approximately 75% of the GI tract, tumors within this section account for only approximately 3% of all GI malignancies and 0.6% of all cancers in the United States, making them relatively rare (Siegel et al., 2018). The disease has a slightly higher incidence in men and in African Americans (both men and women). The median age at diagnosis is 66 years. Death rates rise with age; the average age at death related to small bowel cancer is 72 years (Surveillance, Epidemiology, and End Results Program, 2018).

Etiology and Risk Factors

The etiology of most small bowel cancers is unknown, although a number of risk factors and predisposing conditions have been postu-

Figure 7-1. Anatomy of the Small Intestine

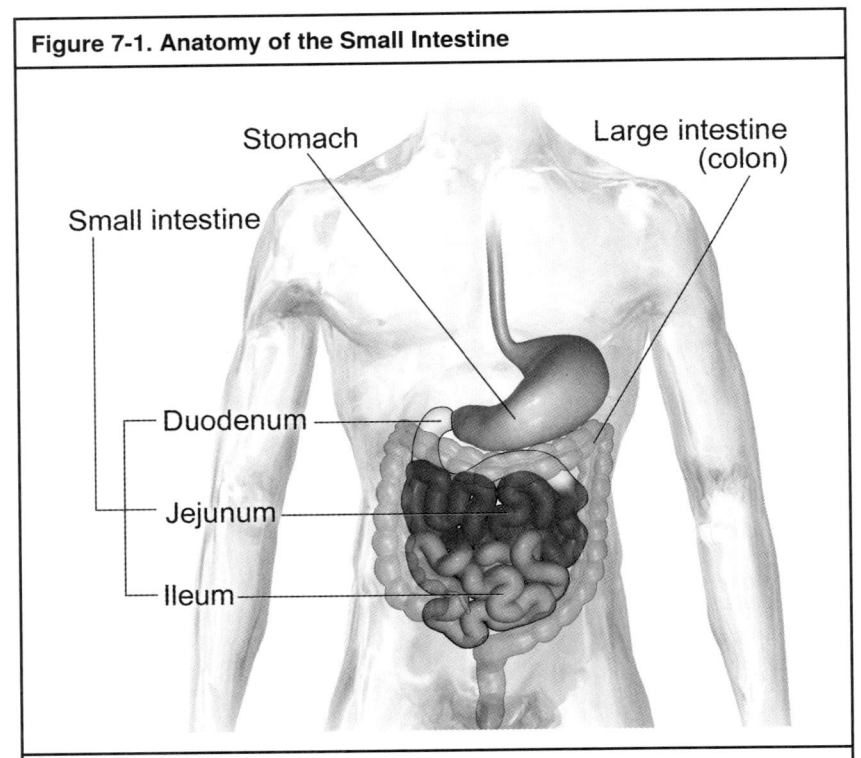

Note. From "Medical Gallery of Blausen Medical 2014," by Blausen.com Staff, 2014, *WikiJournal of Medicine, 1*(2). Retrieved from https://commons.wikimedia.org/wiki/File:Blausen_0817_SmallIntestine_Anatomy.png. Used under the Creative Commons Attribution-ShareAlike 4.0 International (CC BY-SA 4.0) license (https://creativecommons.org/licenses/by-sa/4.0/legalcode).

lated. Benign small intestinal tumors typically are discovered in the fifth and sixth decades of life in the more distal end of the intestine. The most common of these tumors are adenomas, leiomyomas, lipomas, and angiomas, with polypoid adenomas comprising the majority (25%) (Mayer, 2017).

Malignant intestinal adenocarcinomas typically develop from adenomas. Available data suggest an adenoma-to-carcinoma sequence similar to the genetic changes that take place with colorectal cancers. However, this process is not as well documented or understood as that of colorectal cancer (Raghav & Overman, 2013). This type of malignancy is the most common small bowel malignancy (approximately 50%) (Mayer, 2017). Lymphoma (primary or secondary in origin), leiomyosarcomas, and carcinoid tumors comprise the remaining majority of small bowel malignancies (Mayer, 2017).

A strong association exists between an increased risk of adenocarcinoma and several familial cancer syndromes, many of which are linked to specific inherited genetic abnormalities:
- Hereditary nonpolyposis colorectal cancer (HNPCC) is an inherited condition characterized by loss of DNA mismatch repair, which is caused by a germline mutation. Those affected by this condition are at an increased risk for colorectal cancer as well as several other cancers, including adenocarcinomas of the small bowel and endometrium. Similar to colorectal cancer, HNPCC is thought to play a role in approximately 5%–10% of small bowel adenocarcinomas (Overman & Kunitake, 2018).
- Peutz-Jeghers syndrome is a disorder characterized by multiple hamartomatous polyps (tumor-like growths) throughout the intestinal tract and a distinct increased risk for adenocarcinoma in both the large and small bowels (Overman & Kunitake, 2018).
- Familial adenomatous polyposis is associated with a germline mutation in the adenomatosis polyposis coli gene that fosters tumor formation throughout the duodenum and colon. Individuals with this mutation develop numerous polyps in the duodenum, which confer increased risk for transformation into an adenocarcinoma (Overman & Kunitake, 2018).

Additional risk factors, particularly for adenocarcinoma and lymphoma, include chronic inflammation such as that experienced with inflammatory bowel disease (specifically, Crohn disease), chronic immunodeficiency states, and autoimmune disorders, including celiac disease. Modifiable risk factors include dietary choices such as excessive intake of red meat, smoked or cured foods, refined sugars, and alcohol; tobacco use; and obesity (Overman & Kunitake, 2018).

Signs and Symptoms

Signs and symptoms of small bowel cancer are often vague, making this type of cancer difficult to diagnose and creating delays in treatment. Often, radiographic imaging studies appear normal for both the upper and lower GI tract, creating additional delays in diagnosis and treatment (Mayer, 2017). Symptoms include recurrent, unexplained episodes of crampy abdominal pain, anorexia, weight loss, intermittent bouts of intestinal obstruction (specifically in the absence of inflammatory bowel disease or previous abdominal surgery), adults with intussusception, and evidence of chronic intestinal bleeding in the setting of negative conventional and endoscopic examination. Patients presenting with any of these symptoms should be suspicious for small bowel cancer (Chamberlain, Mahendraraj, & Shah, 2015).

Diagnostic Evaluation

No gold standard exists for evaluation of small bowel cancer. All patients should receive a thorough history, physical examination, and basic chemistry and complete blood count analyses. If suspicion of small bowel cancer is high based on symptomology, the options for imaging include plain radiograph, computed tomography [CT] scan, small bowel series, and enteroclysis or endoscopic studies such as wireless capsule endoscopy, push enteroscopy, and double-balloon endoscopy (Chamberlain et al., 2015).

Plain x-ray imaging is of little value unless obstruction is suspected; however, an obstruction does not necessarily confirm the diagnosis of a small bowel cancer (Chamberlain et al., 2015). CT is frequently obtained to evaluate the type of vague abdominal symptoms associated with small bowel cancer. These scans can detect the primary tumor (in many cases) and also are useful in evaluating possible metastatic disease and lymph node involvement (Chamberlain et al., 2015). Upper GI series with small bowel follow-through (UGI/SBFT) may show a lesion, mucosal defect, or intussusception (Chamberlain et al., 2015).

Enteroclysis is a double-contrast radiographic study that is performed by passing a tube into the proximal end of the small bowel and injecting barium and methylcellulose. This technique is considered superior to UGI/SBFT in the detection of malignant small bowel tumors. However, it often fails to reveal flat infiltrating lesions (Chamberlain et al., 2015). CT enterography is an alternative to enteroclysis that is better tolerated by patients because it does not require placement of a nasogastric tube for contrast administration. Instead, patients ingest a large volume of either low-concentration barium or water. This results in distension of the small bowel lumen with a contrast agent that does not interfere with the ability to visualize the lumen and the bowel wall with CT (Chamberlain et al., 2015).

Positron-emission tomography (PET) scanning with the radiotracer 18-fluorodeoxyglucose, particularly integrated PET-CT, may be useful for initial diagnosis, staging, evaluation of the response to treatment, and restaging at the time of suspected disease recurrence (Chamberlain et al., 2015). Standard upper endoscopy is potentially adequate diagnostically; however, it can only reach the proximal end of the duodenum. Therefore, lesions suspected distal to this point would not be visualized (Chamberlain et al., 2015).

Wireless video capsule endoscopy provides a noninvasive method of visualizing the entire small bowel. Its main drawback is that it does not allow for tissue sampling. Additionally, this procedure should not be performed in patients with a suspected small bowel obstruction, as the capsule may become lodged proximal to the obstruction and require laparotomy for retrieval (Chamberlain et al., 2015).

Enteroscopy involves the passage of a colonoscope or special enteroscope beyond the ligament of Treitz, using push, intraoperative, or double-balloon enteroscopy techniques. The main advantage compared to wireless video capsule endoscopy is the ability to obtain tissue samples and perform therapeutic interventions. However, the procedure is invasive and can be technically challenging, and the required expertise and equipment are not always readily available (Chamberlain et al., 2015).

Histology

Differentiating the various small bowel tumors on light microscopy is typically straightforward, and the results of immunohistochemical or cytometric studies can provide a definite diagnosis. Small bowel cancer is divided into benign and malignant histology. The majority (50%) of small bowel malignancies are adenocarcinomas (Mayer, 2017). The other histologies in the malignant group are lymphomas, carcinoid tumors, and leiomyosarcomas and are treated accordingly.

Clinical Staging

Staging is completed according to the American Joint Committee on Cancer tumor-node-metastasis (TNM) staging system (Coit et al., 2017). This staging only applies to adenocarcinomas. Within this system, five classifications are used to identify a time point when the diagnosis was made and appear as a prefix to the category. These classifications are as follows:
- cTNM—clinical
- pTNM—pathologic
- yc/ypTNM—post-therapy
- rTNM—recurrence/progression post-therapy
- aTNM—autopsy

The T, N, and M categories are used to represent the three main anatomic components of the stage (tumor extension, regional lymph node involvement, and distant metastatic involvement). Additionally, some disease sites use subcategories for more detailed reporting. The following are the prognostic stage groupings for small bowel cancers (Coit et al., 2017):
- Stage 0: Tis N0 M0
- Stage I: T1–2 N0 M0

- Stage IIA: T3 N0 M0
- Stage IIB: T4 N0 M0
- Stage IIIA: Any T, N1 M0
- Stage IIIB: Any T, N2 M0
- Stage IV: Any T, Any N, M1

Prognosis

Prognosis depends on the type of small bowel cancer. Adenocarcinomas of the ileum or jejunum have better five-year survival rates than those of the duodenum. Additionally, the presence of distal node involvement or metastases plays a role in prognosis, with inclusion predicting a less favorable prognosis. Further poor prognostic indicators include positive resection margins, poorly differentiated histology, and the presence of lymph node involvement (Young et al., 2016).

Carcinoid tumors tend to be indolent in nature. The five-year survival rate for people with a GI carcinoid tumor that has not spread to other parts of the body is 65%–90%, depending on tumor location. If the tumor has spread to nearby tissue or regional lymph nodes, the five-year survival rate is 46%–78%. For tumors that have spread to distant areas, the survival rate is 14%–54% (Cancer.Net, 2018).

Sarcoma prognosis varies depending on the size, location of the tumor, mitotic rate, and quality of the resection. A study accessing the Surveillance, Epidemiology, and End Results database from 2002 to 2012 reported on 1,848 patients with small intestine gastrointestinal stromal tumors (GISTs) and reported a five-year survival of 83% (DeMatteo et al., 2013).

Primary GI lymphomas are described as lymphomas with the main volume of disease restricted to the GI tract. The following subtypes of lymphoma are primarily seen in the small bowel: non-Hodgkin lymphoma, diffuse large B-cell lymphoma, enteropathy-associated T-cell intestinal lymphoma, extranodal marginal zone B-cell lymphoma of mucosa-associated lymphoid tissue (MALT), mantle cell lymphoma, and Burkitt and Burkitt-like lymphoma. Hodgkin lymphoma in the GI tract is very rare (Cusack, Overman, & Kunitake, 2018). The prognosis of intestinal lymphomas may differ from lymphomas of lymph node origin. For example, an indolent lymph nodal lymphoma may not be localized and can respond to treatment and then recur in time, whereas MALT and MALT-type lymphomas (also indolent in nature) tend to be more localized at diagnosis and are commonly associated with long-term disease-free survival and cure (Cusack et al., 2018).

Treatment

Much like prognosis, the treatment of small bowel cancer is largely dependent on the disease type and stage. Therefore, treatment will be reviewed according to the type of small bowel cancer.

Adenocarcinomas

For adenocarcinomas of local-regional tumors, wide segmental surgical resection is the recommended treatment. Surgical resection of the mesentery (a fold of the peritoneum that attaches the stomach, small intestine, pancreas, spleen, and other organs to the posterior wall of the abdomen) allows for clearance of both the primary and regional nodes at risk for metastases. Further, surgical resection offers important staging information that affects decisions regarding the need for adjuvant therapy. It is important to note, however, that adequate mesenteric resection may be limited by the proximity of the nodes or tumor to the superior mesenteric artery. Tumors that involve the first two portions of the duodenum necessitate a pancreaticoduodenectomy. For tumors involving the distal ileum, a right colectomy with resection of the ileocolic artery and regional lymph nodes is recommended (Raghav & Overman, 2013).

As these types of cancer are rare, few studies are available that address the efficacy of chemotherapy. However, when recommended, adjuvant therapy often comprises chemotherapy regimens similar to those used to treat colon cancer. These include oxaliplatin-based regimens such as FOLFOX (folinic acid, 5-fluorouracil, and oxaliplatin) or FOLFIRI (folinic acid, 5-fluorouracil, and irinotecan), or the use of oxaliplatin with capecitabine (CAPOX) (ACS, 2018b). When the tumor cannot be removed via surgery, radiation therapy becomes another option, most often with the goal of pain relief (ACS, 2018c).

Because of the paucity of randomized trials comparing various chemotherapy regimens, no standard first-line chemotherapy approach exists for patients with advanced small bowel adenocarcinoma. Similar to the use of adjuvant chemotherapy, systemic chemotherapy for patients with advanced small bowel adenocarcinoma has been based on treatment principles established for metastatic colorectal cancer (ACS, 2018b).

Molecular profiling targeted therapies and immunotherapies have not been widely explored; therefore, much of the use is based on indications for colorectal cancers. However, in May 2017, the U.S. Food and Drug Administration approved pembrolizumab for treatment of a variety of advanced solid tumors. This included small bowel adenocarcinomas that were microsatellite instability high or mismatch repair deficient and had progressed after previous treatment, with no further acceptable alternative treatment options (Le et al., 2017).

Carcinoid Tumors

Carcinoid tumors of the small bowel are prone to metastasize, even when smaller than 2 cm in size. Because of this tendency, most surgeons recommend a wide en bloc resection to include the mesentery and adjacent lymph nodes for a small bowel carcinoid of any kind (Cusack et al., 2018). As carcinoid metastases tend to be vascular in nature, hepatic arterial embolization is an option as a palliative technique in patients with hepatic metastases who are no longer candidates for surgical resection. The response rates associated with bland embolization or chemoembolization, as measured by either a decrease in hormonal secretion or radiographic regression, generally are greater than 50%; however, the duration of response can be brief, ranging from 4 to 24 months (Cusack et al., 2018). The role of systemic therapy with metastatic carcinoid tumors is not well outlined. Standard chemotherapy agents have minimal response rates and are generally not recommended, despite location of the primary site. Somatostatin analogs can be useful in controlling the hormonal symptoms resulting from carcinoid syndrome but have a very limited ability to reduce tumor burden (Cusack et al., 2018).

Sarcomas

Sarcomas of the small intestine fall into two main groups: GISTs, which comprise more than 85% of all sarcomas arising within the GI tract, and all other soft tissue sarcomas that arise from other sites, such as leiomyosarcoma, fibrosarcoma, liposarcoma, Kaposi sarcoma, and angiosarcoma. These are classified as "non-GIST" GI sarcomas (Cusack et al., 2018).

GISTs and leiomyosarcomas can appear morphologically similar; however, clearly distinguishing one from the other is of utmost importance, as the treatment is markedly different. The majority of GISTs express mutations in a specific tyrosine kinase receptor (KIT), while the remainder lack this mutation but express a platelet-derived growth factor receptor alpha (PDGFRA) instead (Cusack et al., 2018).

For all GI sarcomas (GISTs and non-GISTs) that are localized with possible negative margins and minimal morbidity, surgical resection remains the initial treatment of choice. The use of en bloc segmental resection with tumor-free margins is preferred over peritumoral resection. To avoid leakage of the tumor, it is critical that the pseudocapsule of the tumor is not disrupted during the resection. If laparoscopic surgery is performed, the tumor should be removed using a specimen retrieval bag (such as the Endo Catch™ pouch) to prevent tumor leakage or seeding of adjacent sites (Cusack et al., 2018).

When GISTs are borderline resectable or advanced in nature, the first-line treatment is an inhibitor of those two receptors (KIT and PDGFRA). Imatinib mesylate (Gleevec®) is the medication of choice.

For patients who are imatinib refractory, sunitinib (Sutent®) or regorafenib (Stivarga®) may be alternate choices (Mayer, 2017).

Lymphoma

Lymphoma of the small intestine typically is initially treated via surgical resection. Some treatments involve postoperative radiation; however, the favored course is to follow surgery with three cycles of systemic chemotherapy. One caveat is that sometimes the disease can be so widespread at the time of diagnosis that complete surgical resection is not possible. If systemic chemotherapy is used as further treatment, patients are at high risk for bowel perforation (Mayer, 2017).

Clinical Trials Influencing Current Treatment

Because of the rarity of small bowel cancers, fewer clinical trials exist than for other GI cancers. However, within the subtypes of small bowel cancer, some types are more common than others (i.e., adenocarcinoma, GIST), and more trials tend to be available. Healthcare providers and patients can view a complete list of current trials at https://clinicaltrials.gov.

Nursing Care

Patients diagnosed with any type of cancer have significant physical and emotional challenges ranging from depression and anxiety to difficulty dealing with treatment and adverse side effects. Depending on the type and stage of small bowel cancer and the type and intensity of treatment, nursing care is wide ranging.

Prevention

Currently, no prevention methods are known for most cases of small bowel cancer. Because smoking may increase the risk of this cancer, risk may be reduced by either never starting smoking or by smoking cessation. Additionally, maintaining a healthy diet high in fruits and vegetables and low in red meat and alcohol and leading an active lifestyle can reduce the risk of developing these types of cancer (ACS, 2018a). People with a genetic predisposition for the development of certain cancers, such as those with familial adenomatous polyposis, HNPCC, or Peutz-Jeghers syndrome (discussed previously), should be considered for genetic testing and follow more stringent screening recommendations (ACS, 2018a).

Surveillance

No guidelines for post-treatment surveillance are available from the American Society of Clinical Oncology, the National Comprehensive Cancer Network®, or the European Society for Medical Oncology for adenocarcinomas of the small bowel. Because of the rarity of this disease and other types of small bowel cancers, many clinicians follow guidelines for surveillance on colorectal cancers. Surveillance and follow-up appointments are decided by the treating oncologist and often based on National Comprehensive Cancer Network guidelines for similar cancers (Overman & Kunitake, 2018).

Survivorship

Patients who have undergone adjuvant therapy will benefit from a cancer survivorship program for surveillance for cancer recurrence and late effects. Patients should receive education on the purpose of survivorship care and important survivorship issues, such as depression and anxiety. Nurses who are able to identify patients who are experiencing altered mood (depressed or anxious) and provide the necessary support (referral to psychosocial services) will afford patients the tools to have a better quality of life. Additional education regarding preventive strategies, such as smoking cessation, routine cancer screenings, healthy diet, and increased physical activity, is important to discuss to decrease risk of recurrence. Further, it is crucial for patients to maintain a relationship with a primary care physician who will be available to care for the routine medical problems that may arise after treatment. Communication between providers is essential to the continued care of cancer survivors and improves the overall quality of life.

Summary

Small bowel cancers are often diagnosed in advanced stages because of their vague symptoms and can vary in cell types, making treatment difficult. Advanced adenocarcinomas of the small bowel are treated with the same chemotherapy used to treat metastatic colorectal cancer, with poor overall response. However, if the disease is identified in the early stages, the five-year survival rate can be as high as 50% and largely depends on the specific type of small bowel cancer and extent of disease at time of treatment (Overman & Kunitake, 2018). As a result, an interprofessional team approach is recommended to ensure proper diagnosis and treatment. Oncology nurses are at the forefront of care and can provide education and information to help advocate for these patients. Educating patients on clinical trials is an important aspect of moving promising treatment options from the bench to the bedside and can provide patients an opportunity for better outcomes.

References

American Cancer Society. (2018a, February 8). Can small intestine cancer (adenocarcinoma) be prevented? Retrieved from https://www.cancer.org/cancer/small-intestine-cancer/causes-risks-prevention/prevention.html

American Cancer Society. (2018b, February 8). Chemotherapy for small intestine cancer (adenocarcinoma). Retrieved from https://www.cancer.org/cancer/small-intestine-cancer/treating/chemotherapy.html

American Cancer Society. (2018c, February 8). Radiation therapy for small intestine cancer (adenocarcinoma). Retrieved from https://www.cancer.org/cancer/small-intestine-cancer/treating/radiation-therapy.html

American Cancer Society. (2018d, February 8). What is a small intestine cancer? Retrieved from https://www.cancer.org/cancer/small-intestine-cancer/about/what-is-small-intestine-cancer.html

Cancer.Net. (2018, August). Neuroendocrine tumor of the gastrointestinal tract: Statistics. Retrieved from https://www.cancer.net/cancer-types/neuroendocrine-tumor-gastrointestinal-tract/statistics

Chamberlain, R.S., Mahendraraj, K., & Shah, S.A. (2015). Cancer of the small bowel. In V.T. DeVita Jr., T.S. Lawrence, & S.A. Rosenberg (Eds.), *DeVita, Hellman, and Rosenberg's cancer: Principles and practice of oncology* (10th ed., pp. 734–744). Philadelphia, PA: Wolters Kluwer Health.

Coit, D.G., Kelsen, D., Tang, L.H., Erasmus, J.J., Gerdes, H., & Hofstetter, W.L. (2017). Small intestine. In M.B. Amin (Ed.), *AJCC cancer staging manual* (8th ed., pp. 221–234). Chicago, IL: Springer.

Cusack, J.C., Jr., Overman, M.J., & Kunitake, H. (2018, April 27). Treatment of small bowel neoplasms. In D.M.F. Savarese (Ed.), *UpToDate*. Retrieved October 12, 2018, from https://www.uptodate.com/contents/treatment-of-small-bowel-neoplasms

DeMatteo, R.P., Ballman, K.V., Antonescu, C.R., Corless, C., Kolesnikova, V., von Mehren, M., ... Kouros, O. (2013). Long-term results of adjuvant imatinib mesylate in localized, high-risk, primary gastrointestinal stromal tumor: ACOSOG Z9000 (Alliance) intergroup phase 2 trial. *Annals of Surgery, 258,* 422–429. https://doi.org/10.1097/SLA.0b013e3182a15eb7.

Le, D.T., Durham, J.N., Smith, K.N., Wang, H., Bartlett, B.R., Aulakh, L.K., ... Diaz, L.A., Jr. (2017). Mismatch repair deficiency predicts response of solid tumors to PD-1 blockade. *Science, 357,* 409–413. https://doi.org/10.1126/science.aan6733

Mayer, R.J. (2017). Upper gastrointestinal tract cancers. In D.L. Longo (Ed.), *Harrison's hematology and oncology* (3rd ed., pp. 542–550). New York, NY: McGraw-Hill.

Overman, M.J., & Kunitake, H. (2018, May 4). Epidemiology, clinical features, and types of small bowel neoplasms. In D.M.F. Savarese (Ed.), *UpToDate*. Retrieved October

15, 2018, from https://www.uptodate.com/contents/epidemiology-clinical-features-and-types-of-small-bowel-neoplasms

Raghav, K., & Overman, M.J. (2013). Small bowel adenocarcinomas—Existing evidence and evolving paradigms. *Nature Reviews Clinical Oncology, 10,* 534–544. https://doi.org/10.1038/nrclinonc.2013.132

Siegel, R.L., Miller, K.D., & Jemal, A. (2018). Cancer statistics, 2018. *CA: A Cancer Journal for Clinicians, 68,* 7–30. https://doi.org/10.3322/caac.21442

Surveillance, Epidemiology, and End Results Program. (2018). Cancer stat facts: Small intestine cancer. Retrieved from https://seer.cancer.gov/statfacts/html/smint.html

Young, J.I., Mongoue-Tchokote, S., Wieghard, N., Mori, M., Vaccaro, G.M., Sheppard, B.C., & Tsikitis, V.L. (2016). Treatment and survival of small-bowel adenocarcinoma in the United States: A comparison with colon cancer. *Diseases of the Colon and Rectum, 59,* 306–315. https://doi.org/10.1097/DCR.0000000000000562

ND
Index

The letter f after a page number indicates that relevant information appears in a figure; the letter t, in a table.

A

abdominoperineal resection (APR), 9
ablation procedures
 for neuroendocrine tumors, 130
adenocarcinoma
 colorectal. *See* colorectal adenocarcinoma
 esophageal. *See also* esophageal cancer
  etiology and risk factors for, 42–43
  prevention of, 60
 gastric, 75
  and proximal polyposis of the stomach, 73
 of small bowel
  clinical staging of, 179–180
  etiology of, 176
  prognosis for, 180
  risk factors for, 177
  treatment of, 181
adjuvant chemoradiation for gastric cancer, 78
adjuvant chemotherapy for colorectal cancer, 11–12, 18–19
adventitia of esophageal wall, 40, 42

aflatoxin B_1 and liver cancer, 143
AFP-L3 fraction in hepatocellular carcinoma, 145
alcohol intake and esophageal cancer, 60
alpha-1 antitrypsin deficiency and hepatocellular carcinoma, 155
alpha-fetoprotein (AFP) testing for hepatocellular carcinoma, 143–145, 160
American Joint Committee on Cancer (AJCC) staging system for liver cancer, 145, 146
ampulla of Vater, 141
anal cancer, 1–29
 clinical staging of, 8–9
 diagnostic evaluation of, 7
 etiology and risk factors for, 5–6
 histology of, 8
 human papillomavirus and, 5–6, 8, 16, 23
 incidence and epidemiology of, 3
 metastatic, 13
 nursing care for, 19–21
 overview of, 1

postoperative management of, 10–12
preoperative management of, 10
prevention of, 23
prognosis for, 21–22
signs and symptoms of, 6
surveillance for, 26
survivorship with, 27–28
treatment of, 9–19
 chemotherapy for, 14–15
 guidelines for, 18
 immunotherapy for, 16, 19
 for metastatic disease, 13
 radiation therapy for, 16–18
 surgical, 9–12
 targeted therapy for, 15, 17t
anemia
 Fanconi, and esophageal cancer, 61
 due to gastric cancer, 73
anorexia-cachexia syndrome due to colorectal cancer, 20
antiangiogenic factor for gastric cancer, 80
antiemetic regimens with esophageal cancer, 56

187

anti–epidermal growth
factor receptor
(anti-EGFR) for gastric
cancer, 79–80
anti-HER2 for gastric
cancer, 79–80
antinausea medication
with esophageal cancer, 56
anti–vascular endothelial growth factor
(anti-VEGF) for gastric
cancer, 79–80
appendix, neuroendocrine tumors of, 119
ascites
  due to colorectal cancer, 20
  due to gastric cancer, 74
aspiration pneumonia
  due to esophageal cancer, 45
aspirin
  and colorectal cancer, 22
  and esophageal cancer, 60
atezolizumab for colorectal cancer, 19

B

back pain due to pancreatic cancer, 97
Barcelona Clinic Liver
  Cancer (BCLC) staging system, 145–146
barium swallow for
  esophageal cancer, 45
Barrett's esophagus (BE),
  43, 60, 61
bevacizumab
  for colorectal and anal
    cancer, 17*t*
  for gastric cancer, 80
bile duct cancer, 157–170
  clinical staging of, 161–162
  diagnostic evaluation of, 159–160
  distal, 141
    histology of, 161

staging of, 161, 162
surgical treatment of, 163
etiology and risk factors
  for, 157–158
extrahepatic, 141
  incidence and epidemiology of, 157
  radiation therapy for, 166
  staging of, 162
high-risk assessment
  (screening and
  genetic testing) for, 168
hilar (Klatskin tumor), 141, 163
histology of, 160–161
incidence and epidemiology of, 157
intrahepatic (perihilar), 141
  clinical staging of, 162
  vs. hepatocellular carcinoma, 145
  histology of, 145
  incidence and epidemiology of, 142, 157
  surgical treatment of, 163
nursing care for, 167
prevention of, 168
prognosis for, 167–168
signs and symptoms of, 158–159
surveillance for, 168–169
survivorship with, 169–170
treatment of, 162–167
  chemotherapy for, 165
  clinical trials influencing, 167
  guidelines for, 167
  immunotherapy for, 166
  radiation therapy for, 166
  surgical, 162–164
bile leaks with biliary
  tract cancers, 164

biliary drainage
  for bile duct cancers, 163
  for pancreatic cancer, 102
biliary tract, 141, 142*f*
biliary tract cancers, 157–170
  clinical staging of, 161–162
  diagnostic evaluation of, 159–160
  etiology and risk factors
    for, 157–158
  high-risk assessment
    (screening and
    genetic testing) for, 168
  histology of, 160–161
  incidence and epidemiology of, 157
  metastatic, 165
  nursing care for, 167
  prevention of, 168
  prognosis for, 167–168
  signs and symptoms of, 158–159
  surveillance for, 168–169
  survivorship with, 169–170
  treatment of, 162–167
    chemoradiation for, 165
    chemotherapy for, 165
    clinical trials influencing, 167
    guidelines for, 167
    immunotherapy for, 166
    radiation therapy for, 166
    surgical, 162–164
  types of, 141
biomarkers
  for colorectal carcinoma, 15
  for pancreatic cancer, 99
bland embolization
  for liver cancer, 148

Index   **189**

for small bowel carcinoid tumors, 182
Bloom syndrome and esophageal cancer, 61
body mass index and gallbladder cancer, 158
and gastric cancer, 72
bowel obstruction due to colorectal cancer, 20
bowel pattern changes with colorectal cancer, 27
BRAF mutation and colorectal cancer, 24
BRCA1/2 mutations and pancreatic cancer, 96, 104
bridging therapies for liver cancer, 147

C

CA 19-9
  in biliary tract cancers, 160
  in pancreatic cancer, 99
cancer-specific immune response in gastric cancer, 79
capecitabine
  for anal cancer, 14–15
  for biliary tract cancers, 165
  for colorectal carcinoma, 11
  for gastric cancer, 77, 79
  for pancreatic cancer, 103, 104
capecitabine and oxaliplatin (CAPOX)
  for pancreatic cancer, 104
  for small bowel adenocarcinoma, 181
capecitabine and temozolomide (CAPTEM)
  for neuroendocrine tumor, 128

carboplatin
  for esophageal cancer, 50
  for gastric cancer, 79, 80
carcinoembryonic antigen (CEA)
  in biliary tract cancers, 160
  in colorectal cancer, 25–26
  in gastric cancer, 74
carcinoid crisis, 127, 128, 132
carcinoid heart disease, 126–127, 132, 133
carcinoid syndrome
  clinical presentation of, 114, 119
  diagnostic evaluation of, 120
  nursing care for, 132
  preoperative management of, 127
  telotristat ethyl for, 129
carcinoid tumors
  classification of, 111–112, 116*t*–117*t*
  etiology of, 113
  gastric, 115–118, 116*t*–117*t*
  of small bowel, 176
  prognosis for, 180
  treatment of, 183
cardiovascular disease after thoracic radiation, 63
catenin beta 1 (*CTNNB1*) mutations and biliary tract cancers, 157
CDKN2A mutations and pancreatic cancer, 96
cecum, neuroendocrine tumors of, 119
celiac plexus block for pancreatic cancer, 97
cell adhesion protein E-cadherin (*CDH1*) gene in gastric cancer, 75, 87
cetuximab
  for colorectal adenocarcinoma, 15, 17*t*
  for gastric cancer, 80

checkpoint inhibitors in esophageal cancer, 48
"chemobrain," 79
chemoembolization for small bowel carcinoid tumors, 182
chemoradiation
  for anal cancer, 14–15
  for biliary tract cancers, 165
  for colorectal carcinoma, 10, 16–17
  for esophageal cancer, 50–51
  for gastric cancer, 77, 78–79, 80–81
  for pancreatic cancer, 102, 104
chemotherapy
  for biliary tract cancers, 165
  for colorectal and anal cancer, 10, 11–12, 13–15, 14*t*, 18–19
  for esophageal cancer, 48, 56
  for gastric cancer, 77, 78–79
  for liver cancer, 147, 150–151
  for neuroendocrine tumor, 128
  for pancreatic cancer, 102, 103–104
  for small bowel adenocarcinoma, 181
Child-Pugh score for liver cancer, 146
cholangiocarcinoma, 157–170
  clinical staging of, 161–162
  diagnostic evaluation of, 159–160
  distal, 141
  histology of, 161
  staging of, 161, 162
  surgical treatment of, 163
  etiology and risk factors for, 157–158
  extrahepatic, 141

incidence and epidemiology of, 157
radiation therapy for, 166
staging of distal, 162
high-risk assessment (screening and genetic testing) for, 168
histology of, 160–161
incidence and epidemiology of, 157
intrahepatic (perihilar), 141
clinical staging of, 162
vs. hepatocellular carcinoma, 145
histology of, 145
incidence and epidemiology of, 142, 157
nursing care for, 167
prevention of, 168
prognosis for, 167–168
signs and symptoms of, 158–159
surveillance for, 168–169
survivorship with, 169–170
treatment of, 162–167
chemotherapy for, 165
clinical trials influencing, 167
guidelines for, 167
immunotherapy for, 166
radiation therapy for, 166
surgical, 162–164
cholangitis, primary sclerosing, and biliary tract cancers, 158, 167
cholecystectomy
for gallbladder cancer, 163
for neuroendocrine tumor, 126
cholecystitis in gallbladder cancer, 158, 163, 168

cisplatin
for biliary tract cancers, 165
for esophageal cancer, 48, 50, 56
for gastric cancer, 79, 85
for neuroendocrine tumor, 128
for pancreatic cancer, 104
cobimetanib for colorectal cancer, 19
coitus, painful, with colorectal cancer, 27
colitis with colorectal and anal cancer
radiation-induced, 18
ulcerative, 5
colon, neuroendocrine tumors of distal, 119
colon cancer. *See also* colorectal adenocarcinoma
clinical staging of, 8
defined, 1
preoperative management of, 10
surgical treatment of, 9
colonic polyps and colorectal cancer, 5
colonoscopy, screening, 22
colorectal adenocarcinoma, 1–29
biomarkers for, 15
clinical staging of, 8
with deficient mismatch repair, 11
diagnostic evaluation of, 6–7
etiology and risk factors for, 3–5, 4t
familial syndromes associated with, 3, 4t, 23–25
high-risk assessment (screening and genetic testing) for, 23–25
histology of, 7
incidence and epidemiology of, 2–3
location of, 1, 2f

metastatic, 12–13, 15, 20
with microsatellite instability, 11, 16, 19, 21, 23–25
nursing care for, 19–21
overview of, 1
postoperative management of, 10–12
preoperative management of, 10
prevention of, 22
prognosis for, 21
signs and symptoms of, 6
surveillance for, 25–26
survivorship with, 26–28
treatment of, 9–19
chemotherapy for, 10, 11–12, 13–15, 14t, 18–19
clinical trials influencing current, 18–19
guidelines for, 18
immunotherapy for, 15–16, 17t, 19
liver-directed, 12
for metastatic disease, 12–13
radiation therapy for, 10, 16–18
surgical, 9–12
targeted therapy for, 15, 17t
complete clinical response in esophageal cancer, 50–51
computed tomography (CT)
of neuroendocrine tumors, 121
of pancreatic cancer, 98
concurrent chemoradiation therapy
for esophageal cancer, 50–51
for gastric cancer, 80
constipation due to opioids for colorectal cancer, 21
coronary artery disease after thoracic radiation, 63

Crohn disease and colorectal cancer, 5
cytopenia due to chemotherapy for anal cancer, 15

D

deficient mismatch repair (dMMR), colorectal adenocarcinoma with, 11, 19, 23–25
depression with colorectal cancer, 27
dermatitis, radiation, with esophageal cancer, 56
descarboxyprothrombin in hepatocellular carcinoma, 145
diabetes and pancreatic cancer, 96
diagnostic laparoscopy for pancreatic cancer, 99, 102
diarrhea
  in carcinoid syndrome, 120
  due to chemotherapy for colorectal carcinoma, 13
  after gastrectomy, 85
  due to neuroendocrine tumor, 115
diet
  and colorectal cancer, 5, 21, 27
  after esophagectomy, 53, 57
  with gastric cancer, 72, 84–85, 86, 88
  with neuroendocrine tumor, 126, 132–133
differentiation of neuroendocrine tumor, 123, 124t
distal colon, neuroendocrine tumors of, 119
distal pancreatectomy with splenectomy, 102

docetaxel
  for esophageal cancer, 48
  for gastric cancer, 79
doxorubicin drug-eluting beads for liver cancer, 148
dumping syndrome
  after esophagectomy, 54, 55t
  after gastrectomy, 84, 85
duodenal neuroendocrine tumors, 116t–117t, 119
duodenum, 175, 176f
dysphagia due to esophageal cancer, 44, 46, 56

E

emesis with esophageal cancer, 56
endoluminal therapy for esophageal cancer, 51
endoscopic mucosal resection (EMR)
  for esophageal cancer, 51, 59
  for gastric cancer, 76, 81
endoscopic submucosal dissection (ESD) for gastric cancer, 76, 81
endoscopic ultrasound (EUS)
  of esophageal cancer, 45–46
  of gastric cancer, 75–76
  of pancreatic cancer, 98
endoscopic ultrasound–guided fine needle aspiration (EUS-FNA) of pancreatic cancer, 98–99
endoscopy of esophageal cancer, 45
enhanced recovery after surgery (ERAS) model after esophagectomy, 53
enteral tube feeding with esophageal cancer, 57–58

enterochromaffin cells, 112, 113
enteroclysis of small bowel cancer, 178
enteroscopy of small bowel cancer, 179
environmental factors and colorectal cancer, 5
epidermal growth factor receptor (EGFR) in colorectal carcinoma, 15, 17t
epidural catheter after esophagectomy, 53
epirubicin, cisplatin and 5-fluorouracil (ECF)
  for esophageal cancer, 48
  for gastric cancer, 78
epirubicin for gastric cancer, 79
erectile dysfunction with colorectal cancer, 27
erlotinib
  for gastric cancer, 80
  for pancreatic cancer, 104
esophageal adenocarcinoma (EAC). See also esophageal cancer
  etiology and risk factors for, 42–43
  prevention of, 60
esophageal anastomotic leak, 53
esophageal anastomotic stricture, 54–55, 55t
esophageal cancer, 39–66
  anatomy of esophagus and, 39–42
  clinical staging of, 46–47, 64
  complete clinical response in, 50–51
  diagnostic evaluation of, 45–46
  etiology and risk factors for, 42–44
  vs. gastric cancer, 64–65, 65t

high-risk assessment (screening and genetic testing) for, 61
incidence and epidemiology of, 42
metastatic, 47, 48, 61
nursing care for, 56–59
  communication in, 59
  enteral tube feeding in, 57–58
  nutrition in, 57
  physical activity in, 58–59
overview of, 39
prevention of, 60–61
prognosis for, 59
signs and symptoms of, 44–45, 44t
sites of, 39–42, 40t, 41f
surveillance for, 62
survivorship with, 62–64
treatment of, 47–56
  chemotherapy for, 48, 56
  concurrent chemoradiation for, 50–51
  endoluminal therapy for, 51
  immunotherapy for, 48–49
  palliative, 55–56
  radiation therapy for, 49–50, 56–57
  surgical, 51–55, 55t
  trimodality therapy for, 47
esophageal stent, 56
esophageal wall, 40–42
esophagectomy, 51–55
  adverse events of, 53–55, 55t
  approaches for, 51–52
  defined, 51
  postoperative course after, 52–53
  preoperative evaluation for, 52
  preoperative teaching for, 52

quality of life after, 62–64
esophagitis, radiation, 57
esophagogastroduodenoscopy (EGD) for gastric cancer, 75, 88
esophagojejunal anastomosis after gastrectomy, 84
esophagojejunostomy for gastric cancer, 82
esophagus
  anatomy of, 39–42, 40t, 41f
  Barrett's, 43, 60, 61
etoposide for neuroendocrine tumor, 128
everolimus for neuroendocrine tumor, 128
external beam radiation therapy (EBRT)
  for gastric cancer, 80
  for liver cancer, 151, 152

F

familial adenomatous polyposis (FAP)
  and colorectal adenocarcinoma, 3, 4t, 23–25
  and small bowel cancer, 177
familial intestinal gastric cancer, 73
Fanconi anemia and esophageal cancer, 61
fatigue with gastric cancer, 73, 85
fertility preservation with radiation therapy, 17–18
fine needle aspiration (FNA) for esophageal cancer, 45–46
18-fluorodeoxyglucose positron-emission tomography (^{18}FDG-PET scan)
  of hepatocellular carcinoma, 144

of neuroendocrine tumors, 121–122
of small bowel cancer, 178
fluoropyrimidines
  for biliary tract cancers, 165
  for colorectal carcinoma, 10, 11–12, 13, 14t, 19
  for pancreatic cancer, 103
5-fluorouracil (5-FU)
  for anal cancer, 14, 17
  for biliary tract cancers, 165
  for colorectal carcinoma, 11–12, 14t
  for esophageal cancer, 48, 50
  for gastric cancer, 77, 79
  for liver cancer, 150
  for neuroendocrine tumor, 128
  for pancreatic cancer, 103, 104
  for small bowel adenocarcinoma, 181
flushing due to neuroendocrine tumor, 114–115
FOLFIRINOX regimen for pancreatic cancer, 104
FOLFIRI regimen for small bowel adenocarcinoma, 181
FOLFOX regimen
  for colorectal carcinoma, 11–12
  for pancreatic cancer, 104
  for small bowel adenocarcinoma, 181
FOLFOX4 regimen for liver cancer, 150
folinic acid
  for pancreatic cancer, 104
  for small bowel adenocarcinoma, 181

foregut neuroendocrine tumors
  classification of, 111, 116t–117t
  of duodenum, 116t–117t, 119
  of pancreas, 116t–117t, 118–119
  signs and symptoms of, 115–119
  of stomach, 115–118, 116t–117t
functional imaging modalities for neuroendocrine tumors, 121–122

G

gallbladder, 141, 157
gallbladder cancer, 157–170
  clinical staging of, 161–162
  diagnostic evaluation of, 159–160
  etiology and risk factors for, 157–158
  high-risk assessment (screening and genetic testing) for, 168
  histology of, 160–161
  incidence and epidemiology of, 157
  nursing care for, 167
  prevention of, 168
  prognosis for, 167–168
  signs and symptoms of, 158–159
  surveillance for, 168–169
  survivorship with, 169–170
  treatment of, 162–167
    chemotherapy for, 165
    clinical trials influencing, 167
    guidelines for, 167
    immunotherapy for, 166
    radiation therapy for, 166
    surgical, 162–164
gallium scan of neuroendocrine tumors, 122
gallstones
  and biliary tract cancers, 157, 159
  with somatostatin analogs, 125–126
gamma counter (Neoprobe) for neuroendocrine tumor, 127
gastrectomy
  partial, 81
  proximal subtotal, 83
  total, 81–85
gastric adenocarcinoma, 75
  and proximal polyposis of the stomach, 73
gastric cancer, 71–89
  classification of, 71, 75
  diagnostic evaluation of, 74–76
    clinical staging in, 75–76, 76f
    endoscopic ultrasound for, 75
    histology for, 75
    laboratory tests in, 74
    physical examination in, 74
  diffuse, 75
  hereditary, 73, 75, 87
  vs. esophageal cancer, 64–65, 65t
  etiology and risk factors for, 71–73
  hereditary (familial), 73
  incidence and epidemiology of, 71
  interprofessional team management of, 64
  intestinal, 75
  familial, 73
  linitis plastica form of, 75, 76, 82
  metastatic, 74, 76–77, 82
  noncardia vs. cardia, 75
  nursing care for, 85–86
  prevention of, 87
  prognosis for, 86–87
  Siewert classification of, 64–65, 65t
  signs and symptoms of, 73–74
  staging of, 64, 75–77, 77f, 82
  surveillance for, 87–88
  survivorship with, 88
  treatment of, 76–85
    chemoradiation for, 77, 78–79, 80–81
    chemotherapy for, 77, 78–79
    immunotherapy for, 79–80
    radiation therapy for, 80–81
    strategy for, 76–77
    surgical, 81–85
gastric carcinoids, 115–118, 116t–117t
gastric fullness due to gastric cancer, 73–74
gastric neuroendocrine tumors, 115–118, 116t–117t
gastric outlet obstruction (GOO) due to pancreatic cancer, 97–98
gastric pouch reconstruction, 83
gastric resection, 77, 81–85
gastrin cells, 112
gastrinomas, 116t–117t, 118
gastroesophageal junction (GEJ)
  cancer of, 71, 75, 81, 87
  defined, 40, 65
  and esophagectomy, 52
  HER2 expression at, 48
  measurement of, 39
  and Siewert classification, 65, 65t
gastroesophageal reflux disease (GERD)
  and esophageal adenocarcinoma, 42, 43, 60, 61

after esophagectomy, 54, 55*t*
due to gastric cancer, 73
gastrointestinal (GI) bleeding due to gastric cancer, 73
gastrointestinal stromal tumors (GISTs) of small intestine, 180, 182–183
gastrointestinal (GI) symptoms after gastrectomy, 84
gastroparesis after esophagectomy, 55, 55*t*
gastrostomy tube with esophageal cancer, 58
gefitinib for gastric cancer, 80
gemcitabine
 for biliary tract cancers, 165
 for pancreatic cancer, 103, 104
gender and gastric cancer, 72–73
glucagonomas, 116*t*–117*t*, 118
glucose monitoring with pancreatic cancer, 103
gray (Gy), 49

H

hand-foot syndrome due to chemotherapy for colorectal carcinoma, 13
Helicobacter pylori and gastric cancer, 72
hemochromatosis, genetic, and hepatocellular carcinoma, 155
hepatectomy for cholangiocarcinoma, 163
hepatic artery embolization
 for neuroendocrine tumor, 130–131
 for small bowel carcinoid tumors, 182

hepatic metastases
 of colorectal cancer, 12–13, 20
 of gastric cancer, 74
 of neuroendocrine tumor, 114, 126, 130–131
hepatic resection, 146–150
hepatitis B virus (HBV)
 and cholangiocarcinoma, 158
 and liver cancer, 143, 144, 154
hepatitis C virus (HCV)
 and cholangiocarcinoma, 158
 and liver cancer, 143, 144, 154
hepatobiliary cancers. *See* biliary tract cancers; liver cancer
hepatocellular carcinoma (HCC), 142–156
 clinical staging of, 145–146
 defined, 141
 diagnostic evaluation of, 143–145
 etiology and risk factors for, 142–143
 fibrolamellar, 145
 high-risk assessment (screening and genetic testing) for, 155
 histology of, 145
 incidence and epidemiology of, 142
 vs. intrahepatic cholangiocarcinoma, 145
 vs. metastatic liver disease, 144
 nursing care for, 153–154
 prevention of, 154–155
 prognosis for, 154
 signs and symptoms of, 143
 surveillance for, 155
 survivorship with, 155–156

treatment of, 146–153
 chemotherapy for, 150–151
 clinical trials influencing, 153
 guidelines for, 152–153
 immunotherapy for, 152
 liver transplantation for, 147, 148, 149
 radiation therapy for, 151–152
 surgery and minimally invasive procedures for, 146–150
HER2
 in biliary tract cancer, 167
 in esophageal cancer, 48–49
hereditary diffuse gastric cancer (HDGC), 73, 75, 87
hereditary nonpolyposis colorectal cancer (HNPCC)
 and bile duct cancer, 158, 163, 168
 and colorectal adenocarcinoma, 3, 4*t*
 and small bowel cancer, 177
hindgut neuroendocrine tumors, 111, 116*t*–117*t*, 119
Howel-Evans syndrome and esophageal cancer, 61
human papillomavirus (HPV) and anal cancer, 5–6, 8, 16, 23
5-hydroxyindoleacetic acid (5-HIAA) in carcinoid syndrome, 120

I

ileocecal valve sparing with neuroendocrine tumor, 127

ileum, 175, 176f
  neuroendocrine tumors of, 119
imatinib mesylate (Gleevec) for small bowel sarcomas, 182
immunosuppression with gastric cancer, 85
immunotherapy
  for biliary tract cancers, 166
  for colorectal and anal cancer, 15–16, 17t, 19
  for esophageal cancer, 48–49
  for gastric cancer, 79–80
  for liver cancer, 152
  for pancreatic cancer, 105
  for small bowel adenocarcinoma, 181
infertility due to radiation therapy for colorectal and anal cancer, 17–18
inflammatory bowel disease and colorectal cancer, 5
insulinoma, 116t–117t, 118
intensity-modulated radiation therapy (IMRT)
  for esophageal cancer, 49
  for pancreatic cancer, 104
interprofessional management of neuroendocrine tumor, 125
intestinal decompression after gastrectomy, 84
intestinal lymphoma, 176
  prognosis for, 180
  risk factors for, 177
  treatment of, 183
intraductal papillary mucinous neoplasms (IPMNs), 95, 100
intravenous (IV) access with esophageal cancer, 56

iodine-131 metaiodobenzylguanidine (^{131}I-MIBG) scan of neuroendocrine tumor, 129
irinotecan
  for colorectal carcinoma, 13, 14t
  for esophageal cancer, 48
  for gastric cancer, 79
  for pancreatic cancer, 104
  for small bowel adenocarcinoma, 181
irreversible electroporation of neuroendocrine tumor, 130
islet cell(s), 118
islet cell tumors, 112, 118

J

Jackson-Pratt drain with biliary tract cancers, 164
jaundice
  due to gallbladder cancer, 158, 159
  due to pancreatic cancer, 97
jejunal feeding tube (J-tube) for gastric cancer, 83
jejunojejunostomy for gastric cancer, 83
jejunostomy tube feeding
  after esophagectomy, 53
  after gastrectomy, 84
  with pancreatic cancer, 103
jejunum, 175, 176f
  neuroendocrine tumors of, 119
juvenile polyposis syndrome, 3, 4t

K

keratosis, nonepidermolytic palmoplantar, and esophageal cancer, 61

Ki-67 proliferative index of neuroendocrine tumor, 123, 124t
KIT receptor in sarcomas of small intestine, 182
Klatskin tumor, 141, 163
KRAS mutations
  in biliary tract cancers, 157
  in colorectal adenocarcinoma, 15
  in pancreatic cancer, 96
Kulchitsky cells, 112, 113

L

lamina propria of esophageal wall, 40–41
lanreotide for neuroendocrine tumor, 125, 132
leiomyosarcoma of small bowel, 176, 182
leucovorin
  for liver cancer, 150
  for pancreatic cancer, 103, 104
lifestyle factors and colorectal cancer, 22, 27
Li-Fraumeni syndrome and esophageal cancer, 61
linitis plastica, 75, 76, 82
liver, 141
liver cancer, 142–156
  Child-Pugh score for, 146
  clinical staging of, 145–146
  defined, 141
  diagnostic evaluation of, 143–145
  etiology and risk factors for, 142–143
  high-risk assessment (screening and genetic testing) for, 155
  histology of, 145
  incidence and epidemiology of, 142

metastatic, 147
Model for End-Stage Liver Disease for, 147
nursing care for, 153–154
prevention of, 154–155
prognosis for, 154
signs and symptoms of, 143
surveillance for, 155
survivorship with, 155–156
treatment of, 146–153
  bridging therapies for, 147
  chemotherapy for, 147, 150–151
  clinical trials influencing, 153
  guidelines for, 152–153
  immunotherapy for, 152
  liver transplantation for, 147, 148, 149
  radiation therapy for, 151–152
  surgery and minimally invasive procedures for, 146–150
types of, 141
liver-directed treatment
  for colorectal adenocarcinoma, 12
  for neuroendocrine tumor, 129–131
liver failure with liver cancer, 149
liver metastases
  of colorectal cancer, 12–13, 20
  of gastric cancer, 74
  of neuroendocrine tumor, 114, 126, 130–131
liver transplantation
  for cholangiocarcinoma, 163
  for liver cancer, 147, 148, 149
  for neuroendocrine tumor, 128

lower esophageal sphincter, 40
lymphadenectomy for gastric cancer, 77, 82, 83
lymphatic mapping for neuroendocrine tumor, 127
lymphoma of small bowel, 176
  prognosis for, 180
  risk factors for, 177
  treatment of, 183
Lynch syndrome, 3, 4t, 23–25

M

magnetic resonance cholangiopancreatography of biliary tract cancers, 159
magnetic resonance imaging (MRI)
  of neuroendocrine tumors, 121
  of pancreatic cancer, 98
malabsorption
  after esophagectomy, 64
  with neuroendocrine tumor, 126
  due to pancreatic cancer, 97
matuzumab for gastric cancer, 80
metaiodobenzylguanidine (MIBG) for neuroendocrine tumor, 129
metastasis
  of biliary tract cancers, 165
  of colorectal and anal cancer, 12–13, 15, 20
  of esophageal cancer, 47, 48, 61
  of gastric cancer, 74, 76–77, 82
  of liver cancer, 147
  of neuroendocrine tumor, 114, 115, 124, 126, 129, 130–131

of pancreatic cancer, 98, 99, 104
microsatellite instability (MSI)
  colorectal adenocarcinoma with, 11, 16, 19, 21, 23–25
  esophageal cancer with, 61
microwave ablation for liver cancer, 148
midgut neuroendocrine tumors, 111, 116t–117t, 119
minimally invasive procedures for liver cancer, 146–150
mismatch repair–deficient (dMMR) tumors
  of biliary tract, 166
  colorectal, 11, 19, 23–25
mitomycin C for anal cancer, 14, 15, 17
mitotic index of neuroendocrine tumor, 123, 124t
MLH1 and colorectal cancer, 23, 24
Model for End-Stage Liver Disease (MELD), 147
monoclonal antibodies (mAbs)
  for colorectal and anal cancer, 15, 16, 17t, 19
  for esophageal cancer, 48–49
  for gastric cancer, 79–80
MSH2 and colorectal cancer, 23, 24
MSH6 and colorectal cancer, 23, 24
mucosa-associated lymphoid tissue (MALT) lymphomas of small bowel, 180
mucosa of esophageal wall, 40–41
mucositis due to chemotherapy for colorectal carcinoma, 13

Index   197

multikinase inhibitor for liver cancer, 150
multiple endocrine neoplasia type 1 (MEN1) and neuroendocrine tumors, 113
multivisceral transplantation for neuroendocrine tumor, 128
muscularis mucosae of esophageal wall, 41
muscularis propria of esophageal wall, 40, 41–42

N

nab-paclitaxel for pancreatic cancer, 104
NanoKnife for neuroendocrine tumor, 130
napabucasin for pancreatic cancer, 106
nasogastric tube
 after gastrectomy, 84
 with pancreatic cancer, 103
nausea with gastric cancer, 74, 85
neoadjuvant chemoradiation
 for colorectal carcinoma, 16–17, 19
 for esophageal cancer, 50–51
 for gastric cancer, 78–79, 81
 for locally advanced rectal cancer, 19
 for pancreatic cancer, 102
neoadjuvant chemotherapy
 for colorectal cancer, 11
 for gastric cancer, 78–79
 for pancreatic cancer, 102
neuroendocrine tumors (NETs), 111–135
 biochemical evaluation of, 120

characteristics of, 111
classification of, 111–112
clinical presentation of, 113–115, 116t–117t
clinical staging of, 124
defined, 111
diagnostic evaluation of, 120–123
 guidelines for, 122–123
differentiation of, 123, 124t
etiology and risk factors for, 113
foregut, 111, 115–119, 116t–117t
 of duodenum, 116t–117t, 119
 of pancreas, 116t–117t, 118–119
 of stomach, 115–118, 116t–117t
functional, 114–115, 118–119
grade of, 123–124, 124t
hindgut, 111, 116t–117t, 119
histology of, 123–124, 124t
imaging of, 120–123
 CT for, 121
 functional, 121–122
 MRI for, 121
 positron-emission tomography for, 122
 somatostatin receptor scintigraphy for, 122
incidence and epidemiology of, 112–113
Ki-67 proliferative index of, 123, 124t
locations of, 111
metastatic, 114, 115, 124, 126, 129, 130–131
midgut, 111, 116t–117t, 119
mitotic index of, 123, 124t
nonfunctional, 114, 115, 119

nursing care for, 131–134
 for carcinoid crisis, 127, 128, 132
 for carcinoid heart disease, 126–127, 132, 133
 nutrition in, 126, 132–133
 patient resources and advice in, 133–134
 symptom management in, 131–132
overview of, 111–112
prevention of, 134
prognosis for, 134
signs and symptoms of, 113–119
surveillance for, 134
survivorship with, 134–135
treatment of, 125–131
 chemotherapy for, 128
 clinical trials on, 131
 guidelines for, 131
 interprofessional management in, 125
 liver-directed therapy for, 129–131
 metaiodobenzylguanidine for, 129
 peptide receptor radionuclide therapy for, 129
 somatostatin analogs in, 125–126
 surgical, 126–128
 targeted therapy for, 128–129
 transplantation for, 128
neuropathic symptoms due to chemotherapy for colorectal carcinoma, 13–14
neutropenia due to chemotherapy for anal cancer, 15
nivolumab
 for colorectal and anal adenocarcinoma, 16, 17t, 19

for liver cancer, 152
nonalcoholic fatty liver disease and hepatocellular carcinoma, 155
nonsteroidal anti-inflammatory drugs (NSAIDs) and esophageal cancer, 60
NRAS in colorectal adenocarcinoma, 15
nutrition
 with esophageal cancer, 57
 with gastric cancer, 84–85, 86, 88
 with neuroendocrine tumor, 126, 132–133
 with pancreatic cancer, 103
nutritional deficits after esophagectomy, 63–64

O

Oberndorfer, Siegfried, 111
obesity
 and esophageal adenocarcinoma, 42–43, 60
 and gastric cancer, 72
 and hepatocellular carcinoma, 155
 and pancreatic cancer, 96
octreotide for neuroendocrine tumor, 113, 125, 127, 132
octreotide scan of neuroendocrine tumors, 122
odynophagia due to esophageal cancer, 44
Okuda staging system for liver cancer, 145
opioid analgesia for colorectal cancer, 20–21
oral cancer and esophageal cancer, 61
oxaliplatin
 for biliary tract cancers, 165

 for colorectal carcinoma, 11–12, 13–14, 14*t*, 18–19, 27
 for esophageal cancer, 50
 for gastric cancer, 79
 for liver cancer, 150
 for pancreatic cancer, 104
 for small bowel adenocarcinoma, 181

P

paclitaxel
 for esophageal cancer, 48, 50
 for gastric cancer, 79, 80
 for pancreatic cancer, 104
pain after esophagectomy, 53
PALB2 mutations and pancreatic cancer, 96, 104
palliation for esophageal cancer, 55–56
palmar-plantar erythrodysesthesia due to chemotherapy for colorectal carcinoma, 13
palmoplantar keratosis, nonepidermolytic, and esophageal cancer, 61
pancreas, 95, 97
pancreatectomy
 distal, 102
 total, 102
pancreatic cancer, 95–109
 diagnostic evaluation of, 98–101
 biomarkers in, 99
 clinical staging in, 100–101, 101*f*
 CT and MRI for, 98
 diagnostic laparoscopy for, 99, 102
 endoscopic ultrasound–guided fine needle aspiration for, 98–99

 histology in, 99–100
 positron-emission tomography for, 99
 endocrine. *See* neuroendocrine tumors (NETs)
 etiology of, 95–96
 exocrine, 95
 genetic syndromes associated with, 96–97
 incidence and epidemiology of, 95
 and intraductal papillary mucinous neoplasms, 95, 100
 metastatic, 98, 99, 104
 nursing care for, 106
 prevention of, 107
 prognosis for, 106–107
 risk factors for, 96–97
 signs and symptoms of, 97–98
 staging of, 98, 100–101, 101*f*
 surveillance of, 107
 survivorship with, 107–108
 treatment of, 101–106
  chemoradiation for, 102, 104
  chemotherapy for, 102, 103–104
  clinical trials on, 105–106
  guidelines for, 105
  immunotherapy for, 105
  radiation therapy for, 104–105
  surgical, 101–103
pancreatic ductal adenocarcinomas (PDACs), 95–96, 99
pancreatic enzymes, 125, 133
 with biliary tract cancers, 164
pancreatic exocrine insufficiency due to pancreatic cancer, 97
pancreatic leak with biliary tract cancers, 164

Index   199

pancreatic neuroendocrine tumors (PNETs), 116t–117t, 118–119
pancreaticoduodenectomy
  for cholangiocarcinoma, 163
  for pancreatic cancer, 102
panitumumab
  for colorectal adenocarcinoma, 15, 17t
  for gastric cancer, 80
patient education
  for colorectal cancer, 27
  for gastric cancer, 86
  for liver cancer, 156
pembrolizumab
  for biliary tract cancers, 166
  for colorectal adenocarcinoma, 16, 17t, 19
  for esophageal cancer, 61
  for small bowel adenocarcinoma, 181
peptide receptor radionuclide therapy (PRRT) for neuroendocrine tumor, 129
perioperative chemotherapy for gastric cancer, 78
peripheral neuropathy due to chemotherapy for colorectal carcinoma, 13–14, 27
peristalsis, 41–42
peritoneal carcinomatosis due to gastric cancer, 74
Peutz-Jeghers syndrome
  and colorectal cancer, 3, 4t
  and small bowel cancer, 177
pharyngeal cancer and esophageal cancer, 61
physical activity
  and colorectal cancer, 22, 27

and esophageal cancer, 58–59
physical examination for esophageal cancer, 45
platelet-derived growth factor receptor alpha (PDGFRA) in sarcomas of small intestine, 182
platinum for gastric cancer, 79
PMS2 and colorectal cancer, 23, 24
pneumonia, aspiration, due to esophageal cancer, 45
pneumonitis, radiation, with esophageal cancer, 56–57
polyps, colonic, and colorectal cancer, 5
portal vein embolization for biliary tract cancers, 163
positron-emission tomography (PET)
  of hepatocellular carcinoma, 144
  of neuroendocrine tumors, 121, 122
  of pancreatic cancer, 99
  of small bowel cancer, 178
positron-emission tomography–computed tomography (PET-CT)
  of biliary tract cancers, 159
  of small bowel cancer, 178
prepyloric tube with esophageal cancer, 58
primary liver cancer. See liver cancer
primary sclerosing cholangitis (PSC) and biliary tract cancers, 158, 167, 168
programmed cell death protein 1 (PD-1)
  in colorectal and anal cancer, 16, 17t, 19

in liver cancer, 152
programmed cell death protein-ligand 1 (PD-L1) in esophageal cancer, 48
protein induced by vitamin K absence or antagonist II (PIVKA-II) in hepatocellular carcinoma, 145
proton pump inhibitors (PPIs)
  for esophageal cancer, 60
  and neuroendocrine tumors, 113
proton therapy for esophageal cancer, 49–50
pruritus due to pancreatic cancer, 97
pyloric outlet obstruction due to pancreatic cancer, 97

Q

quality of life
  with colorectal cancer, 27
  with esophageal cancer, 62–64

R

radiation dermatitis with esophageal cancer, 56
radiation esophagitis, 57
radiation-induced colitis with colorectal and anal cancer, 18
radiation pneumonitis with esophageal cancer, 56–57
radiation therapy
  for biliary tract cancers, 166
  for colorectal and anal cancer, 10, 16–18
  for esophageal cancer, 49–50, 56–57
  for gastric cancer, 80–81

for liver cancer, 151–152
for pancreatic cancer, 104–105
for small bowel adenocarcinoma, 181
and squamous cell carcinoma of esophagus, 44
radiofrequency ablation (RFA) for liver cancer, 147–148
ramucirumab for esophageal cancer, 48
rectal cancer. *See also* colorectal adenocarcinoma
  clinical staging of, 8
  defined, 1
  incidence and epidemiology of, 2
  locally advanced, 19
  preoperative management of, 10
  surgical treatment of, 9
rectum, neuroendocrine tumors of, 119
regorafenib (Stivarga)
  for colorectal cancer, 17t
  for liver cancer, 150
  for small bowel sarcomas, 183
regurgitation due to esophageal cancer, 45
Roux-en-Y anastomosis for gastric cancer, 82, 83

S

sarcoma of small bowel, 176
  prognosis for, 180
  treatment of, 182–183
serotonin in carcinoid syndrome, 120
sexual dysfunction with colorectal cancer, 27
Siewert classification, 64–65, 65t
signet ring carcinomas, 7

single photon emission computed tomography (SPECT) of neuroendocrine tumors, 122
Sister Mary Joseph nodule, 74
small bowel cancer, 175–185
  adenocarcinomas as
    clinical staging of, 179–180
    etiology of, 176
    prognosis for, 180
    risk factors for, 177
    treatment of, 181
  carcinoid tumors as, 176
    prognosis for, 180
    treatment of, 183
  clinical staging of, 179–180
  diagnostic evaluation of, 178–179
  etiology and risk factors for, 175–177
  histology of, 179
  incidence and epidemiology of, 175
  lymphoma as, 176
    prognosis for, 180
    risk factors for, 177
    treatment of, 183
  nursing care for, 183
  prevention of, 183
  prognosis for, 180
  sarcomas as, 176
    prognosis for, 180
    treatment of, 182–183
  signs and symptoms of, 177
  surveillance for, 184
  survivorship with, 184
  treatment of, 181–183
    for adenocarcinomas, 181
    for carcinoid tumors, 182
    clinical trials influencing, 183
    for lymphoma, 183
    for sarcomas, 182–183
  small intestine, 175, 176f

smokeless tobacco and pancreatic cancer, 96
smoking
  and esophageal cancer, 60
  and pancreatic cancer, 96
somatostatin, 113, 125
somatostatin analogs (SSAs)
  for neuroendocrine tumors, 113, 121–122, 125–126
  for small bowel carcinoid tumors, 182
somatostatinomas, 116t–117t, 119
somatostatin receptors (SSTRs), 113, 121–122
somatostatin receptor scintigraphy of neuroendocrine tumors, 122
sorafenib for liver cancer, 150, 152
splenectomy
  for gastric cancer, 82
  for pancreatic cancer, 102
squamous cell carcinoma (SCC) of esophagus. *See also* esophageal cancer
  etiology and risk factors for, 43–44
  prevention of, 60
staging laparoscopy for gastric cancer, 76
stereotactic body radiation therapy (SBRT)
  for liver cancer, 151
  for pancreatic cancer, 104
stomach, neuroendocrine tumors of, 115–118, 116t–117t
streptozotocin for neuroendocrine tumor, 128
submucosa of esophageal wall, 40, 41
suicide with esophageal cancer, 59

sunitinib (Sutent)
  for neuroendocrine syndrome, 129
  for small bowel sarcomas, 183
surgical treatment
  for biliary tract cancers, 162–164
  for colorectal and anal cancer, 9–12
  for esophageal cancer, 51–55, 55*t*
  for gastric cancer, 81–85
  for liver cancer, 146–150
  for neuroendocrine tumor, 126–128
  for pancreatic cancer, 101–103
  for small bowel cancers, 181, 182
swallow study after gastrectomy, 84
Sweet syndrome, 114

T

targeted therapy
  for colorectal and anal cancer, 15, 17*t*
  for neuroendocrine tumor, 128–129
  for small bowel adenocarcinoma, 181
telotristat ethyl for neuroendocrine tumor, 129, 132
temozolomide for neuroendocrine tumor, 128

thoracic radiation, survivorship after, 63
three-dimensional conformal radiation therapy for pancreatic cancer, 104
thromboembolic disease
  with liver cancer, 149
  with pancreatic cancer, 103
transarterial chemotherapy for liver cancer, 147
transarterial radioembolization for liver cancer, 151–152
trastuzumab
  for biliary tract cancer, 167
  for esophageal cancer, 48
  for gastric cancer, 80
trifluridine-tipiracil for colorectal carcinoma, 14*t*
trimodality therapy for esophageal cancer, 47
tyrosine kinase inhibitors for gastric cancer, 80

U

ulcerative colitis and colorectal cancer, 5

V

vascular endothelial growth factor (VEGF)

  in colorectal carcinoma, 15, 17*t*
vasomotor collapse with neuroendocrine tumor, 127, 132
Verner-Morrison syndrome, 118
VIPomas, 116*t*–117*t*, 118
vomiting
  with esophageal cancer, 39
  with gastric cancer, 85

W

weight loss
  after gastrectomy, 84–85
  due to gastric cancer, 73
Whipple procedure
  for cholangiocarcinoma, 163
  for pancreatic cancer, 102
Whipple triad, 118
wireless video capsule endoscopy of small bowel cancer, 178–179

Y

yttrium-90 (^{90}Y) for liver cancer, 148, 151–152

Z

ziv-aflibercept for colorectal cancer, 17*t*
Zollinger-Ellison syndrome, 114, 115–118

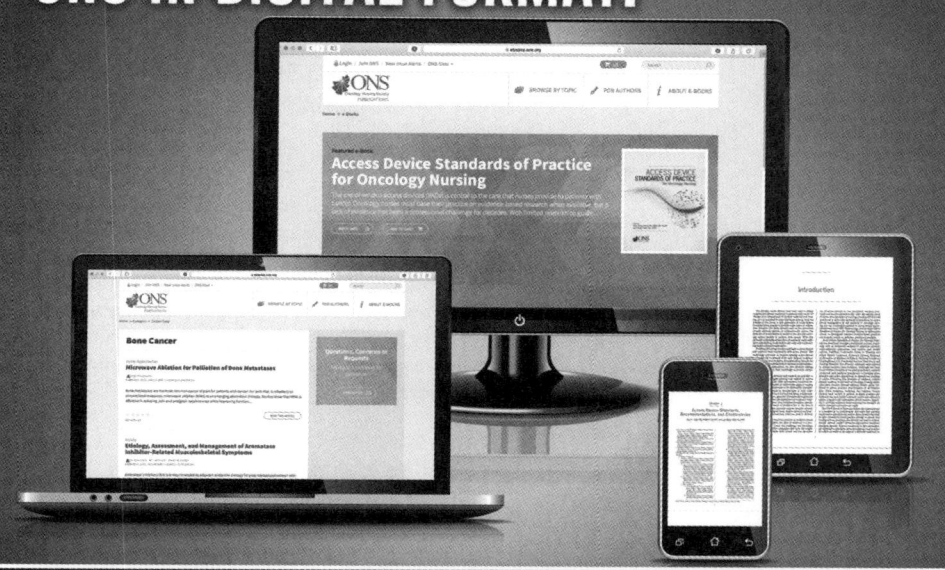

Also From ONS

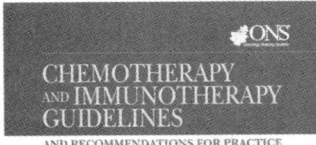

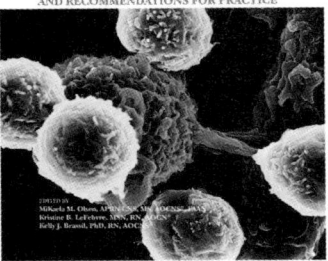

CHEMOTHERAPY AND IMMUNOTHERAPY GUIDELINES AND RECOMMENDATIONS FOR PRACTICE
Edited by M.M. Olsen, K.B. LeFebvre, and K.J. Brassil

Chemotherapy and Immunotherapy Guidelines and Recommendations for Practice is a continuation of the chemotherapy and biotherapy guidelines and features 26 chapters with crucial updates on chemotherapy administration and safe handling, and, in response to the rapid rise of immunotherapy in cancer care, new content on immunotherapy approaches, treatments, and side effects. 2018. 658 pages. Softcover.

ISBN: **9781635930207** • Item: **INPU0684**
E-book available at https://ebooks.ons.org

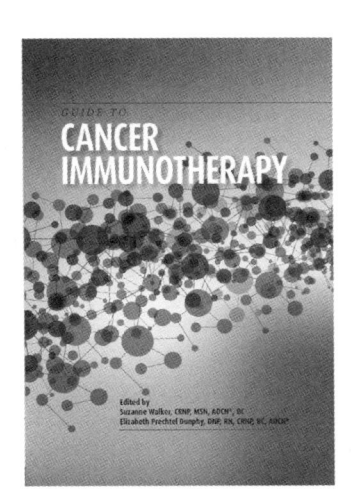

GUIDE TO CANCER IMMUNOTHERAPY
Edited by S. Walker and E.P. Dunphy

Guide to Cancer Immunotherapy was developed by an expert collection of healthcare professionals and nursing leaders to provide nurses with in-depth knowledge on the principles of immunology, cancer and the immune system, and the history of immunotherapy. This foundational work is supported with information on the development of new agents and classes of agents, active immunization, passive/adoptive immunotherapy, combination therapies, biomarkers, and many other topics. 2018. 336 pages. Softcover.

ISBN: **9781635930184** • Item: **INPU0676**
E-book available at https://ebooks.ons.org

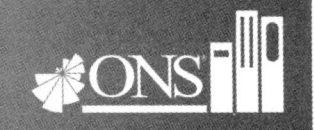

WWW.ONS.ORG/ONS-STORE